Lifeguards of the Jersey Shore

A Story of Ocean Rescue in New Jersey

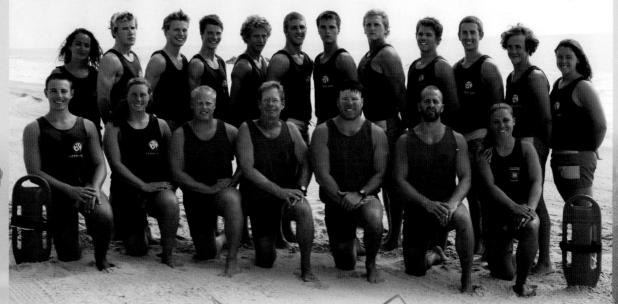

U.S. LIFE SAVING SERVICE

Michael "Spike" Fowler,
Bernard A. Olsen, & Edward B. Olsen

Schiffer Publishing Ltd

4880 Lower Valley Road, Atglen, Pennsylvania 19310

Dedications

I dedicate this work to my family — my wonderful wife Gloria and sons Stephen and David — and I also apologize to my wife for lifeguarding for half a day on our wedding day.

I also wish to acknowledge all the lifeguards, past and present that I have had the honor and privilege of working with.

~ Michael "Spike" Fowler

We dedicate this book to Erik, Laura, Anna, and Mary.

~ Bernard A. and Edward "Ted" Olsen

Map of the Jersey Shore, reproduced with permission of the artist Ann Sader; © 1994. It's available as a poster from Locust Hill Press, P.O. Box 100, St. Stephens Church, VA 23148

Other Schiffer Books on Related Subjects:
Stars of the Jersey Shore: A Theatrical History, 978-0-7643-2719-3, $19.95
The Roaring '20s at the Jersey Shore, 978-07643-3218-0-, $24.99
New Jersey's Southern Shore: An Illustrated History from Brigantine to Cape May Point, 978-0-7643-3009-4, $29.99

Library of Congress Control Number: 2010924845

Designed by Mark David Bowyer
Type set in Isadora / Souvenir Lt BT, KR Down By The Sea

ISBN: 978-0-7643-3491-7
Printed in China

Schiffer Books are available at special discounts for bulk purchases for sales promotions or premiums. Special editions, including personalized covers, corporate imprints, and excerpts can be created in large quantities for special needs. For more information contact the publisher:

Published by Schiffer Publishing Ltd.
4880 Lower Valley Road
Atglen, PA 19310
Phone: (610) 593-1777; Fax: (610) 593-2002
E-mail: Info@schifferbooks.com

For the largest selection of fine reference books on this and related subjects, please visit our web site at:
www.schifferbooks.com
We are always looking for people to write books on new and related subjects. If you have an idea for a book please contact us at the above address.

This book may be purchased from the publisher.
Include $5.00 for shipping.
Please try your bookstore first.
You may write for a free catalog.

In Europe, Schiffer books are distributed by
Bushwood Books
6 Marksbury Ave.
Kew Gardens
Surrey TW9 4JF England
Phone: 44 (0) 20 8392 8585; Fax: 44 (0) 20 8392 9876
E-mail: info@bushwoodbooks.co.uk
Website: www.bushwoodbooks.co.uk

Contents

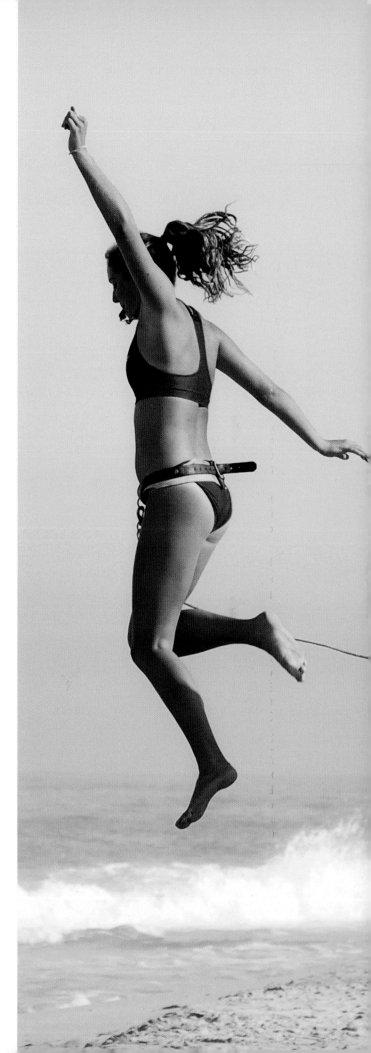

Acknowledgments

We are indebted to the many contributors who made this publication possible.

We thank the following people who gave interviews for their time and resources:

~ Harry Back, Harry "Buzz" Mogck, and Jack Schellenger, Cape May Beach Patrol
~ Captain Sandy Bosacco, Stone Harbor Beach Patrol
~ Andrew Fedick, Monmouth County Park System Lifeguard
~ Steve Healey, Seaside Heights Beach Patrol
~ Harry Hoehn, Allenhurst Beach Patrol
~ Thomas Hoffman, Gateway National Recreation Area
~ Dr. Eugene Leahy, Risden's Beach
~ Don Myers, Long Beach Township Beach Patrol
~ Dave Pearson, Sandy Hook Beach Patrol
~ Howard Rowland, Belmar Beach Patrol
~ B. Chris Brewster, president of the United States Lifesaving Association (for authoring the Foreword)

All the following organizations gave us access to photos and other memorabilia from their private collections, or reviewed the photos and manuscript for us. We are indebted to their sharing of resources:

~ John Angemi, Jr., Director of Avalon Free Library and History Center
~ Olivia Arnone, Newark Museum
~ Bob Bright, Wildwood Historical Society
~ Courtney Caram, photo consultation
~ Ken Child, Avon-by-the-Sea
~ Christopher Connors, Long Beach Township Beach Patrol
~ Bob Dillon, United States Lifesaving Association
~ Dorn's Classic Images
~ Bill Dunn and Conrad Yauch, Sea Girt Lighthouse
~ Joan Ellis, of Middletown
~ Jim Foley, of Point Pleasant
~ Gloria J. Fowler, David Fowler, and Kathleen Olsen, manuscript consultants

~ Stephen Fowler and Andrew J. Olsen, Lifeguard Consultants
~ Paul Goldblatt of Cape May
~ Bob Harris, Mantoloking Beach Association
~ Gordon Hesse, author of *All Summer Long*
~ Dick Johnson and John McCahill, Bradley Beach Beach Patrol
~ Matt Karch, Marlboro High School
~ Heather Halpin, archivist, Heston Collection, Atlantic City Free Public Library
~ Tim Harmon, Sea Girt Beach Patrol
~ Charles Hartl, United States Lifesaving Association
~ Dr. Joseph Jasaitis of Avon
~ Kristin Joson of Ocean City, Maryland, Beach Patrol
~ Nancy Kegelman and George Moss and the Moss Family of Rumson
~ Jess LeVine, Avon-by-the-Sea Lifeguard
~ Robert Longo of Pennsylvania
~ Dale Lonkart, Archivst Librarian, Atlantic Carriage Center
~ Dr. Thomas P. McCann, Sea Isle City Beach Patrol
~ James M. McPherson, Princeton University
~ Fred Miller, Ocean City Beach Patrol and historian
~ Liam Moroney, Monmouth County Historical Association
~ Monmouth County Park System
~ National Archives Still Picture Reference Team, College Park, Maryland
~ Bernard John Olsen and Christian Olsen, research consultants
~ Mary Rasa, Sandy Hook archivist
~ Barbara Reynolds, Squan Village Historical Society
~ Ann Ryan, Sea Girt Public Library
~ John Shaw, reference librarian, New Jersey State Library
~ Robert Stewart, Asbury Park Public Library
~ Don Stine of Asbury Park
~ Beverly Streeter of Belmar
~ George Valente, of Jersey Shore Publications
~ Mary Ware and Bob Watkins, Jr. of Manasquan
~ Kathleen Wells of Ship Bottom
~ Beth Woolley of Long Branch Historical Association
~ Lewis Wyman, Reference Section, Library of Congress, Washington, D.C.

Foreword

For well over a century, intrepid men and women have left the safety of the Jersey Shore to come to the rescue of those imperiled by the mortal dangers of thundering surf and clawing currents. How many panicked faces have these rescuers calmed? How many families have they made whole? How many people who were certain of their own untimely demise have they plucked from the maw of death? No one knows.

A visit to the Jersey Shore on a typical summer day features the lifeguards on their stands, sentinels of the surf, overseeing a casual assembly, where happy, careless fun prevails. Perhaps a lost child is reunited with a parent or a laceration is bandaged. But at every moment, the lifeguard scans for the desperate beachgoer who is unexpectedly, silently imperiled by a current racing away from shore. And at every moment, the lifeguard sits prepared, like a coiled spring that can release itself on command.

In a typical year, over 3,000 rescues from drowning are performed along the Jersey Shore. Some the lifeguard may consider routine, easy. Some unfold in the most arduous conditions imaginable, with multiple victims clawing for life in heavy surf and strong currents. Regardless, the outcome is almost universally the same. A life that was lost is not. The lifeguard returns to the stand. The rescued continue lives uninterrupted by abrupt conclusion.

The lifeguards of the Jersey Shore are part of a tradition dating back to the nineteenth century, when lifesavers rescued the shipwrecked in horrendous storms, day and night, throughout the year, so that others might live. In fact, the very first beach lifeguards in the United States were assigned to patrol the Jersey Shore in the late 1800s and their service continues to this day. The methods and the implements of rescue have changed somewhat, but the ethos is timeless.

Here are the stories of these lifesavers: where they worked, what they accomplished, and how the profession has evolved. They are stories of people who embraced a role in which they would put the safety of others ahead of their own, in fair weather and foul, with a single, simple goal. Lifesaving.

~ B. Chris Brewster, President
United States Lifesaving Association

Preface

*T*he mystique of the ocean has enthralled mankind since time immemorial. With the seas covering about sixty-five percent of the earth's surfaces, it is not surprising the physical proximity of this resource has impacted dramatically on the human condition. Politically, socially, economically and in a host of other areas, the oceans have played a significant role in our evolution. Indeed, the theory that life itself originated in the earth's oceans is still a widely held belief. Rachel Carson writes in her book, *The Sea Around Us*, "when the animals went ashore to take up life on the land, they carried part of the sea in their bodies, a heritage which they passed on to their children and which even today links each land animal with its origins in the ancient sea."

For those who have been exposed to the sea, whether born and raised near its environs or perhaps settled nearby later, there is a magic aura that seems to permeate the soul and lures them back. It becomes a subtle, subjective, and unconscious force that might be classified as a positive addiction. Once the individual has witnessed the wonders of the ocean and its shores they have experienced something they can never forget. Whether it is the smell of the salt air, the sound of the breakers and gulls, the blue green and white froth of the waves or some aggregate thereof, it becomes a mystical lore that hypnotizes and mesmerizes. The land that receives the awesome force of the ocean is a combination of sand, shells, organic matter, living and non-living organisms, sand dunes and shore birds. The beauty of the shore, of course, fits together and compliments the ocean. The sand dunes nestled along long stretches of open space serve a unique environment of flora and fauna. These vary in America from East to West, and from North to South.

In New Jersey, holly, cypress, bayberry, cedar, prickly pear, cactus, goldenrod and beach heather often combine to create a mosaic of beauty that natives simply call "the beach."

In New Jersey, Native Americans of the Lenni-Lenape tribes spent the summer at the sea fishing and gathering shellfish. As early as 1609, it is quite probable that Henry Hudson's sailors enjoyed the ocean and beaches of New Jersey. By the turn of the twentieth century, "sea-bathing" had become popular. As historian Harold F. Wilson writes, "It consisted of wading in the water and jumping joyously up and down in the surf." It is to this environment, replete with its own unique beauty that humans have congregated since early times. Today the shore is no longer merely a seasonal resource as it is enjoyed year round by increasing numbers of people. It is still however, the hot summer months that attendance is highest along the Jersey Shore as visitors have continued to seek relief from the heat and humidity of the hinterland.

Lifeguards of the Jersey Shore: A Story of Ocean Rescue in New Jersey endeavors to trace the origins of this service against the backdrop of the conditions that necessitated its evolution; conditions both natural and man-made. Most significantly, it is an attempt to place in perspective the scope and depth of modern ocean lifeguarding. Finally, it seeks to focus respect and gratitude to those who have made it their vocation to protect the lives of the public from the perils of the sea.

~ Michael Fowler, Bernard A. Olsen,
and Edward B. Olsen
July 2009

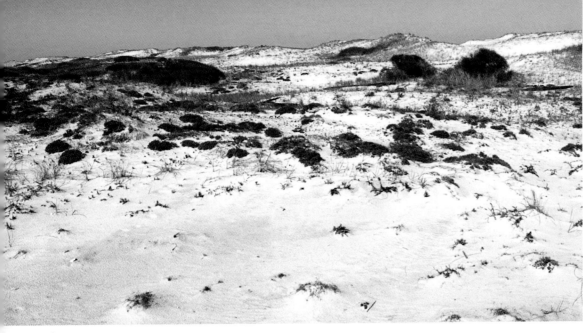

The earliest visitors to the Jersey Shore would have found miles of pristine sand dunes ... as shown here at Island Beach State Park. Some areas had pine forests stretching to the water's edge.

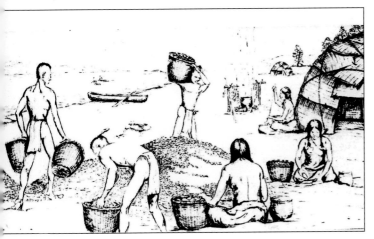

The real first travelers to the Jersey Shore were the Lenni Lenape Indians who came primarily for food, but also to escape the oppressive inland heat, dust, and insects. The tribe would seine the bays and estuaries near the shoreline for the plentiful supplies of fish and shellfish. *Photo courtesy of the Newark Museum.*

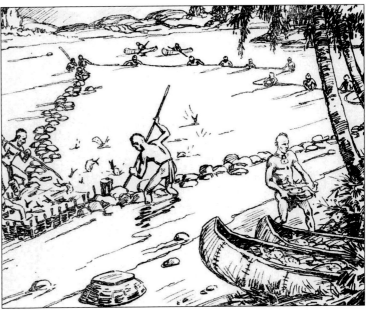

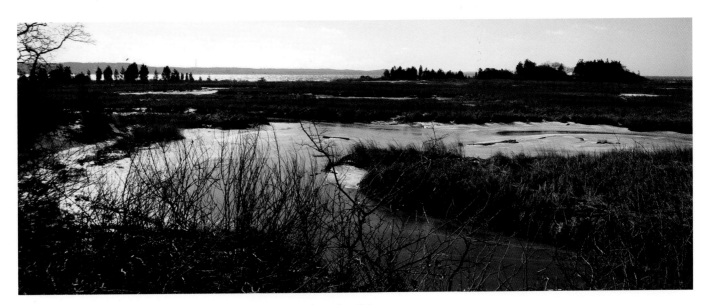

Behind the barrier beaches were bays and estuaries, providing plentiful food supplies for early explorers as well as the Lenni-Lenape Indians.

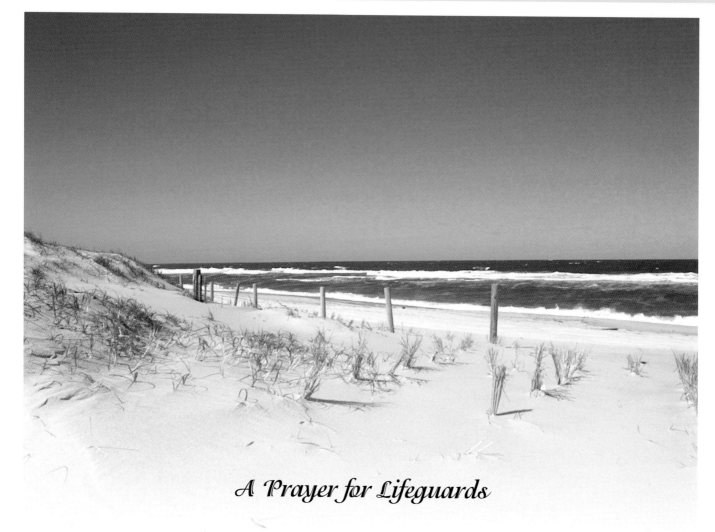

A Prayer for Lifeguards

Oh Lord our God who stills the sea,
Watch o'er these brave ones we do pray thee
Guide those whose vigilance and care
Protect us on the beaches and dare
The roughened waters to bring back
One who ventured far, whose strength is slack.
We beseech thee, Oh lord, that you
Grant them courage, faith, endurance too.
Keeping strong in body, heart, and will
Striving to help with consummate skill
We're grateful and know that in your way
You'll bless, and keep each Lifeguard every day.

~ Beersheba Station, Ocean Grove
July 20, 1984

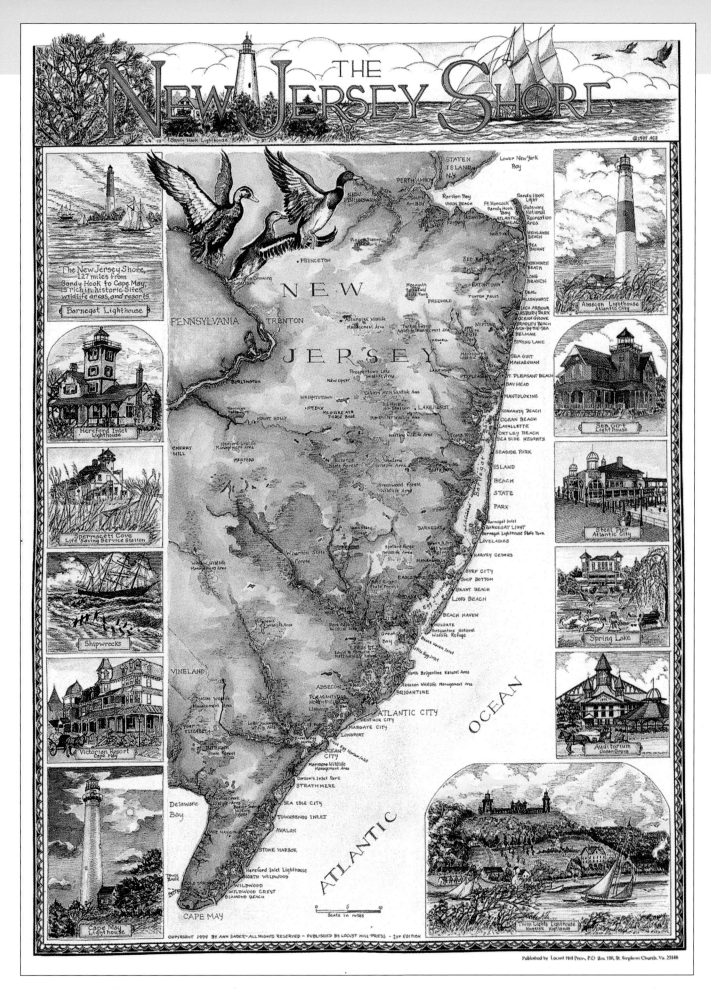

Map of the Jersey Shore. *Courtesy of Ann Sader.*

Chapter One
Life at the Seashore

The wonders of the New Jersey Shore are a fusion of ingredients that offer something for everyone. The foundation upon which everything else rests is the combination of hot summer weather and the beautiful Atlantic Ocean. This translates into a mass exodus of people from the interior to coastal shores of the United States each summer. Indeed, New Jersey alone attracts millions of tourists each year and is considered a national attraction. Belmar as an example has a year round population of 6,000 swelling to over 16,000 during the summer. The transition from a few bathers to crowds submerged in the sea has been a steady and persistent evolution that has no signs of abating. For those familiar with the Jersey Shore during the summer months, it is not uncommon to see beachfronts filled with thousands of people sun tanning, swimming, body-boarding, skim-boarding, surfing, kayaking, and snorkeling. Many of these bathers become mesmerized by the euphoria of the surf with its awesome waves and mysterious currents masking lurking dangers such as rip currents and undertows. The safety of the public is left to a small but dedicated corps of professional lifeguards who assume the responsibility of rescuing would-be victims from drowning in the sea.

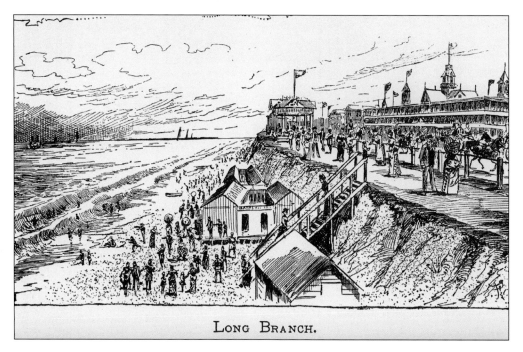

LONG BRANCH.

An 1869 *Long Branch News* editorial warned of the dangers of ocean bathing and commented on the frequent drownings at this resort. By 1880 typical shore literature called for beach surveillance and suggested that measures be taken to protect the public. This drawing shows the bluffs in 1889. *Courtesy of Gustave Kobbe.*

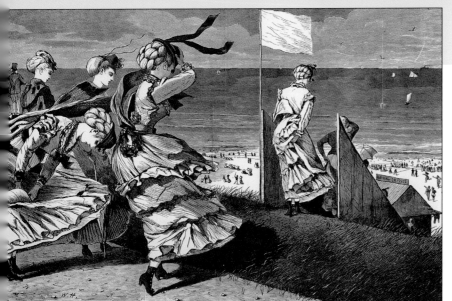

Mixed bathing was strictly forbidden. The men's time often began at dawn and was designated by a red flag while the ladies turn was signaled by a white flag. This practice dated back to 1819 according to Gustave Kobbe. Mrs. Francis Trollope, an early English visitor observed how American ladies "enjoyed ...to taste the briny wave." Proper attire was also expected as elaborate costumes emerged. *Harpers Weekly, August 6, 1870; Courtesy of George H. Moss, Jr.*

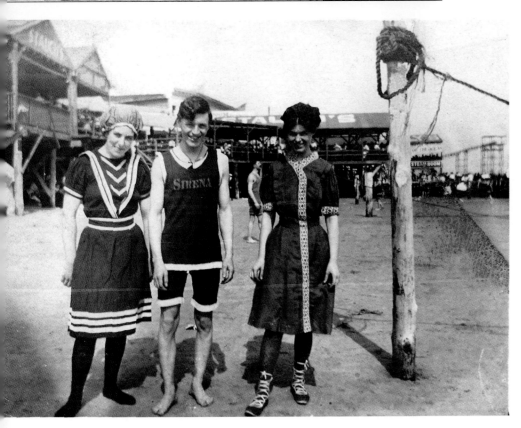

Modesty standards were strictly enforced in the early days of ocean bathing. Police officers were equipped with measuring sticks to make certain hem lengths were not too short. Bathing costumes that became heavy when wet made ocean bathing uncomfortable at best. Here, three bathing beauties pose at Atlantic City. *Courtesy of the Atlantic City Library, Heston Collection.*

This 1844 view shows the early towers and lighthouses constructed in 1828 on Beacon Hill, which is the site of the present day Twin Lights of the Navesink. This hill, the highest on the eastern seaboard eventually became the site of the most powerful lighthouse in America.

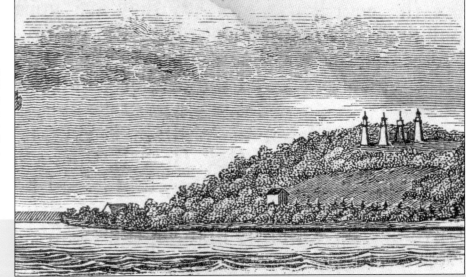

By the mid-nineteenth century, strict bathing rules were introduced. These reflected Victorian values of propriety and grew out of perspectives expressed by local newspapers of the day. An 1868 *New York Daily Tribune* article characterized the beach as a place where all social classes met "for no other purpose than to exhibit oneself."

The article stated the ideal bathing costume for a lady was "delicate rose flannel with pleatings of white, pink hose, straw shoes and a broad brimmed hat of chipped straw tied with a pink flannel bow under the chin." The fashionable man wore, "a tight fitting blue shirt with a white star on the breast or a loose sailor's shirt and trousers handsomely braided."

The winds of change brought an end to the colored flags and segregated bathing. By the last decades of the century, a simple white flag was introduced to announce calm sea conditions. Rules and regulations persisted however, as pamphlets and brochures served as guidelines for prospective ocean bathers. An 1885 booklet, *Summer Days in New Jersey*, warned about the risk of losing one's teeth while bathing and advised the public to run for ten minutes up and down the beach before entering the surf.

Schenck's Guide for "Rules Which Are In Order For Sea Bathers" advised, among other things, not to enter the sea alone, stay in for only three to five minutes, and to defer to the bathing master — the precursor of the modern lifeguard. The perils of the ocean were recognized early on. *Schenck's Guide* continued:

"The full force of the sea is shoreward and if taken off your feet you are thrown on the beach — a frolic in which many indulge. On the other hand, when the tide recedes a miniature maelstrom is formed, termed the 'sea-puss,' being a sort of under-tow, is dangerous, sometimes taking a person out to sea."

A *Long Branch News* editorial read, "It is well if every seaside resort, a corps of men were kept to patrol the beach, sound its waters and place cautionary signals, carrying appliances, for rescuing and restoring the drowning. They might be supported by the corporation of the town, or by hotels and boarding houses, or private subscription." Ocean lifeguarding in New Jersey was about to emerge.

The evolution of the modern ocean lifeguard is linked to the increasing popularity of ocean bathing and swimming. A visit today to a New Jersey beach such as Sandy Hook, Seven Presidents Oceanfront Park, Asbury Park, Belmar, Island Beach State Park, Atlantic City or Cape May on a beautiful, clear, and warm July weekend is a case in point. Several distinguished lifeguard supervisors have reported that the ratio of guards to patrons can be as many as 1:800. These numbers can challenge the most skillful and dedicated ocean rescue crews.

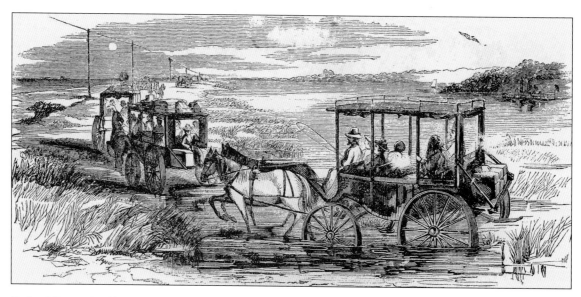

Early visitors arrived by various means, including wide-wheeled carriages, the railroad, and steamships. This view shows transportation south along the beachfront toward Long Branch in 1857. *Frank Leslie's Illustrated Newspaper, August 22, 1857; Courtesy of George H. Moss, Jr.*

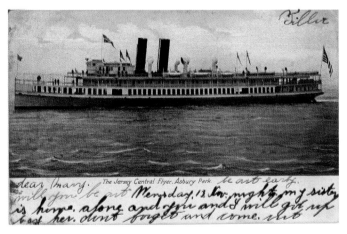

Steamships carried thousands of early travelers to the shore. Shown is the Jersey Central Flyer off Asbury Park.

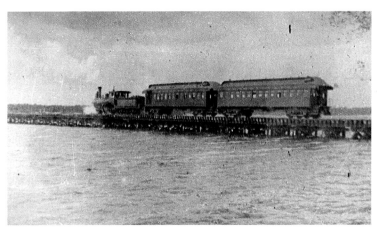

A train carries passengers bound for the shore across the Toms River Bridge to the Seaside resort area circa 1890. *Courtesy of Steve Healey.*

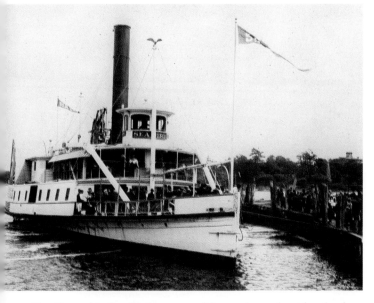

The Steamship *Sea Bird* was one of the most popular side-wheelers along the New York to Red Bank route. At 187 feet, it was one of the largest vessels on this route and ran uninterrupted for sixty years. *Courtesy of George Moss.*

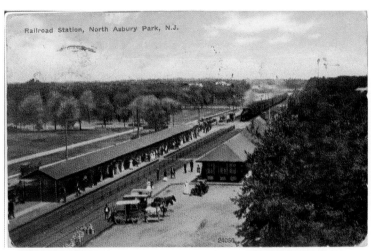

Early travelers to the Jersey Shore also traveled by rail with thousands often arriving daily during the busy summer months. Here a train pulls into the Asbury Park Railroad station in 1911 where guests would be taken by carriage or boat to resorts along Ocean Avenue.

Many of the millions who swim in the ocean each year disregard or are unaware of the hazards of sea bathing. They frequently swim too far off the beach and are swept out in rip currents or what was referred to in the early days as "beyond their depth." When this occurs they seek assistance from lifeguards who willingly risk their own safety to save those in trouble. Jersey shore lifeguards rescue thousands of patrons each season from life-threatening ocean conditions. These staggering statistics suggest the type of demands placed on the modern lifeguard: unpredictable weather conditions, vulnerable and susceptible swimmers, and unwieldy numbers. These combine to challenge the skills of the most accomplished lifeguards who are always ready and willing to pit their skills against some of the Atlantic Ocean's harshest conditions, among the worst of which are the feared nor'easters.

Lifeguards of the Jersey Shore: A Story of Ocean Rescue in New Jersey tells how and why modern ocean lifeguarding emerged in New Jersey. Here is the story from the early lifelines, to constables of the surf, volunteers, bathing masters, to paid lifeguards — each played a role in the foundation for today's highly trained and skilled ocean rescue crews.

Big Sea Day was also referred to as the "Annual Salt Water Day," pictured here in 1916 in
Manasquan. Note the photographers apparently
taking souvenir photos. It was a tradition started
in the mid-1800s and lasted until shortly after
World War I. It started in the Raritan Bay area
and eventually shifted to the Wreck Pond area
of Sea Girt, spreading south into Manasquan.
Typically held the second Saturday in August, the event often led to drunkenness and
debauchery with "hucksters, sharpsters, and
gamblers." Modern revivals of this event have
not brought large crowds as it once did.
Courtesy of Mary Ware.

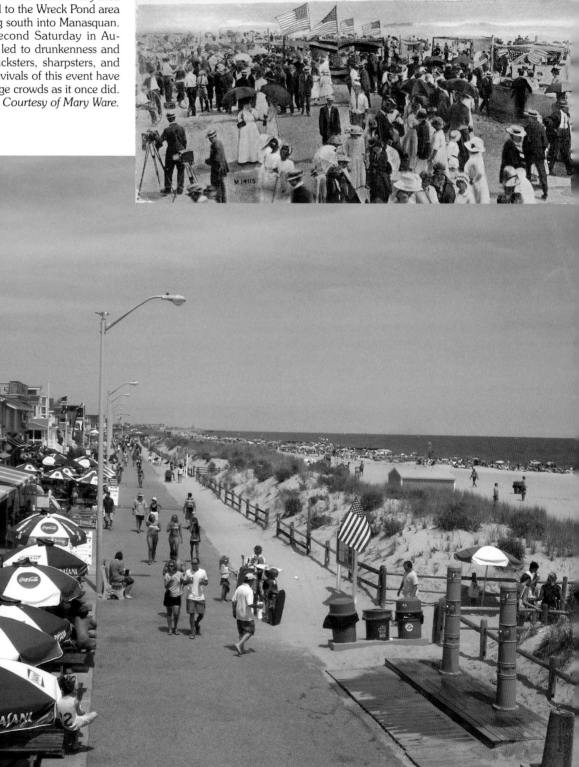

An August 2009 revival of Big Sea Day in Manasquan reveals little of the crowds and festivities the day once
brought. Modern shore communities have little tolerance for noise, drunkenness, gamblers, or hucksters.

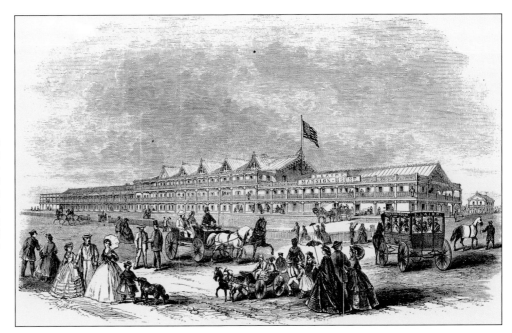

Beautiful and elaborate hotels spanned the shore from Cape May to Long Branch to accommodate the early visitors to shore resorts. Pictured is the Mansion House along Ocean Avenue in Long Branch in 1863. *Frank Leslie's Illustrated Newspaper, August 1, 1863; Courtesy of George H. Moss, Jr.*

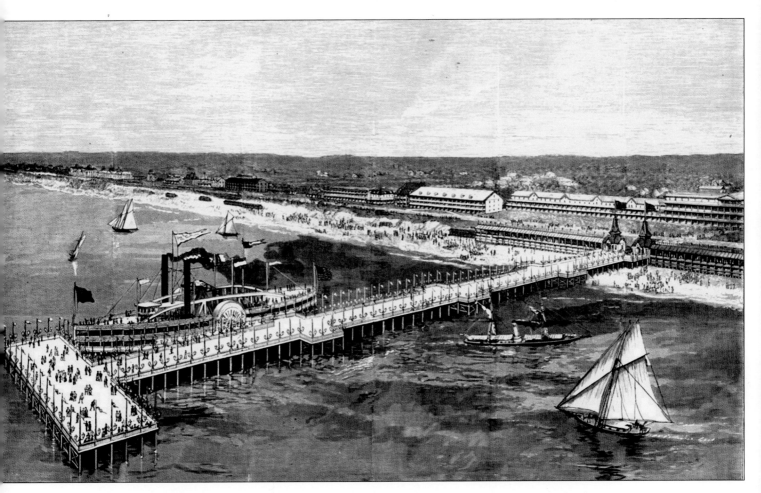

In northern resorts such as here in Long Branch, visitors arrived by the thousands on steamships coming down from New York. *Harpers Weekly, June 21, 1879; Courtesy of George H. Moss, Jr.*

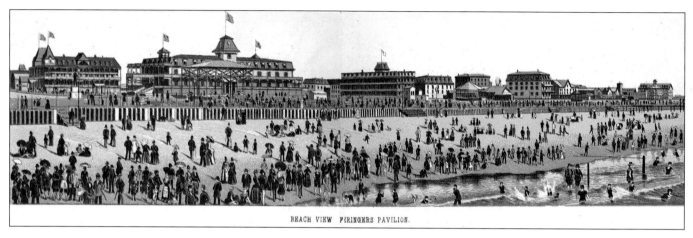

BEACH VIEW PERINGERS PAVILION.

This view of Ocean Grove in the 1890s shows how splashing around changed as the decades of the nineteenth century wore on. It was originally considered a bathing process that was an act of cleanliness designed to increase circulation and restore "healthfulness and vigor." "Buoyance and cheerfulness of spirit" were expected results. Sea bathing was not swimming, but "jumping up and down as the waves came in."

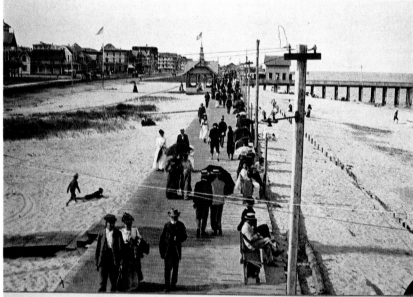

BOARD WALK, OCEAN GROVE.

Leisurely strolls along the boardwalk were a popular pastime in the late 1800s as this 1896 view along the Ocean Grove boardwalk shows. *Courtesy of Don Stine.*

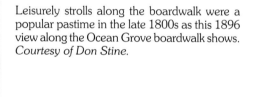

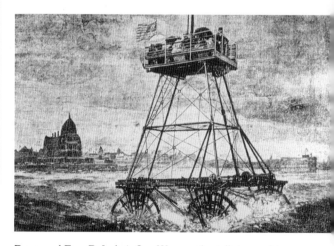

Reverend Ezra B. Lake's Sea Wagon: the tall steam-driven contrivance was designed for use by the Life-Saving Service, but after a demonstration in Ocean City in 1884, was never put into production or use. Dr. Lake was one of the founders of Ocean City. *Courtesy of Fred Miller.*

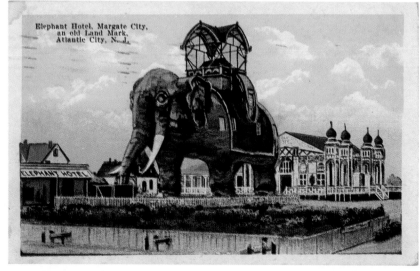

An early Jersey Shore attraction was Lucy, the Margate Elephant. It was constructed in 1881 by James Lafferty from Philadelphia to attract people to his land holdings. Lucy was toured by Woodrow Wilson in 1916; through the years it has been moved, and served as a private residence and hotel. It is now on the National Register of Historic Places.

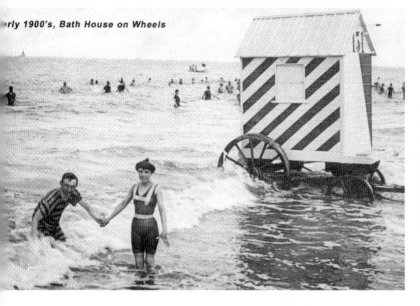

rly 1900's, Bath House on Wheels

Early bathing contrivances such as this bathhouse on wheels were designed to provide both convenience and modesty in the early days of ocean bathing. Modesty was a big legal issue in the early days of seashore bathing and police in Atlantic City were issued measuring sticks to make certain women's suits met minimum length standards. Violators were issued a summons. The heavy woolen suits lasted until the 1940s when rubber and nylon suits were introduced. The rubber suits would eventually split from the effects of the salt water.

An 1890s view of Asbury Park shows lifelines, but no lifeguards or volunteer lifesavers. Large poles were jetted in with fire hoses and linked by the lifelines marking the "safe" bathing areas. A shipwreck sits on shore as a grim reminder of the perils of the sea.

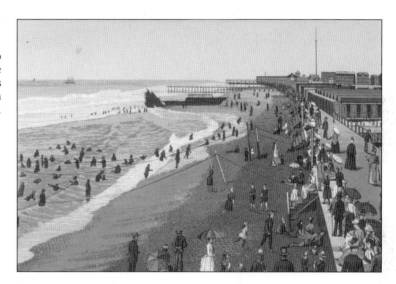

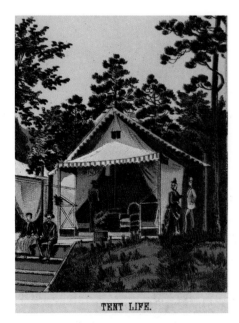

TENT LIFE.

Ocean Grove, the first religious resort on the Jersey Shore, held summer meetings that drew over 10,000 people. The community enforced strict codes of conduct, which included no dancing, card playing, alcohol, tobacco, and driving on Sundays. By 1875 there were six hundred tents; today, there are about one hundred tents that remain.

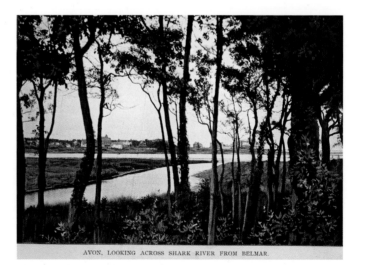

AVON, LOOKING ACROSS SHARK RIVER FROM BELMAR.

The lands comprising Avon-by-the-Sea, formerly Key East, were purchased by Edward Batchelor in 1879 for $45,000. The parcels were originally planned for tobacco farming. When he realized the potential of a quiet and beautiful seaside community, he changed his plans and turned toward real estate development. Most notably, he established the Avon Inn, a Jersey Shore landmark for decades. *Courtesy of Don Stine.*

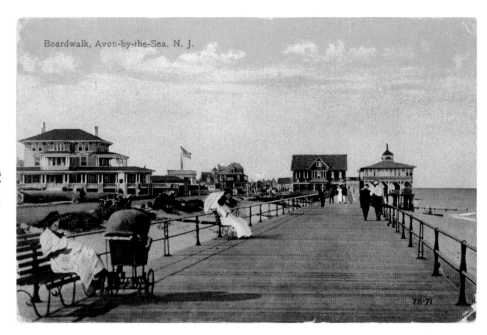

Boardwalk strolls have always been a popular pastime as shown in this 1917 view in Avon-by-the-Sea.

Rescued from Hurricane Donna
Bernard Olsen

Hurricane Donna came ashore on the outer banks of North Carolina impacting the Jersey shore. September 12, 1960 dawned cloudy and humid amidst reports of an impending storm. I hitchhiked down Rumson Road and made my way to Sea Bright early that morning to see what I had been told was impressive surf conditions. Impressive was not the word for it! The waves were the biggest I had ever seen and were the type that body surfers dream of. Huge, rolling sets of surf that promised to give a swimmer the "ride" of his life. After all, I considered myself a veteran ocean swimmer in all of my fourteen years. As I headed to the beach of what was then Edgewater Beach Club, I vividly remember reading about what nineteenth century whalers called a "Nantucket Sleigh Ride." This was the dangerous yet exhilarating race that jettisoned longboats through the ocean at high speeds behind harpooned whales. Somehow, in my youthful delusion of invincibility I was determined to have my own sleigh ride.

I entered the surf and enjoyed my first encounter with a giant "roller." I was strong, in good shape and full of energy. I had broken the first basic rule of swimming: never go in alone. I measured up to the second wave with no problem, thrilled with the awesome power of nature that I had harnessed, or so I thought. I was so fixated with the fun I was having that I didn't notice that fatigue was setting in and the ocean conditions were steadily worsening. The wave sets were getting even bigger and were quickening which is a "red flag" to those who know the surf. Under these conditions, a swimmer cannot recover after riding a wave because the next wave is upon him. This was the situation I found myself in; I couldn't return to shore because I would be pummeled by unrelenting waves and I couldn't swim out beyond the "break." I was at the mercy of the monster I set out to tame.

Time passed like an eternity as I struggled to survive. Time and time again I was driven beneath the raging surf and dragged along the sand. I vividly recall my lungs reaching the bursting point as I somehow miraculously broke the surface for yet one more gulp of air. Surely there must be someone on the beach who could see me but through the mist I saw no one. My thoughts turned to my family, my friends, my school; disconnected by a delirium and some inner knowledge that I was drowning. I prayed for the strength for one last try for the beach when I felt something grab the back of my bathing suit. I looked around and saw the bald head of a man yelling in my ear to do what he said. He told me, at his signal, to break for the beach and that he would be right behind me if I got in trouble. I realized that he was timing the "sets" and I stood a better chance of surviving with him that I did on my own. The sinews of my body ached as I mustered one last burst of energy. I felt sand beneath my feet. Could I have reached safety? The bald headed man screamed at me to keep going and pushed me forward. I finally reached the safety of the beach collapsing in exhaustion. The middle aged man struggled to safety and it was then that I knew that he had put his own life in jeopardy to save mine.

When my mind cleared, I understood that he was the popular lifeguard that my friends and I had swum with many times that summer. His name was Pat, a name I will never forget. It would not be until years later that I would realize that Pat was but one of thousands of dedicated professionals, "sentinels on the sand," who devoted and risked their lives saving people from the perils of the sea.

Chapter Two

Guardians of the Jersey Shore

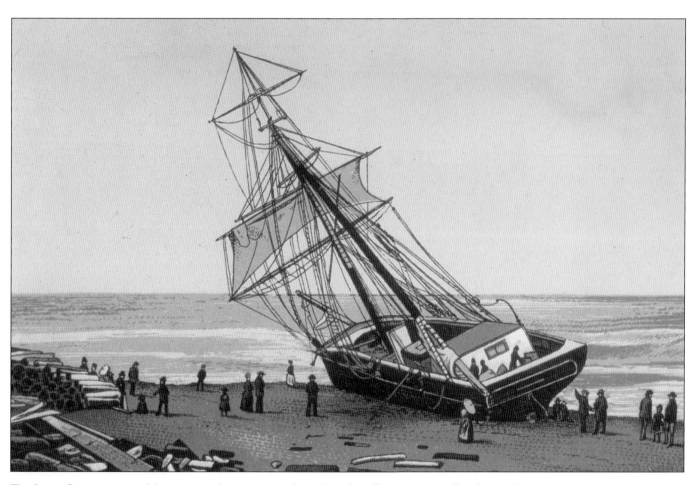

The Jersey Coast was one of the most treacherous regions for early sailors. There was a sandbar that ran the entire length of the New Jersey coast from 300 to 800 yards offshore and had only two feet of water at low tide.

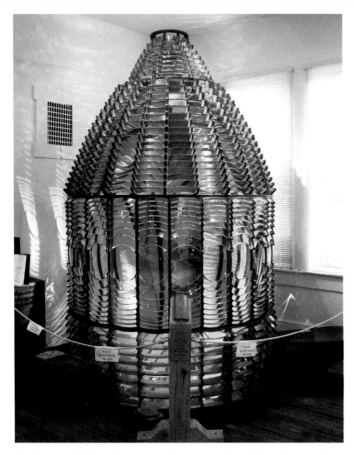

New Jersey Lighthouses

The dangers of the sea were aptly chronicled in 1880 by James H. Merryman, an officer of the Revenue Marine and chief inspector of the board, examining the Life-Saving Service:

"No portion of the ten thousand and more miles of the sea and lake coast-line of the United States, extending through every variety of climate and containing every feature of coast danger to the mariner, can exhibit a more terrible record of shipwrecks than the long stretch of sandy beaches lying between Cape Cod and Cape Hatteras. This region, the New Jersey coast is notoriously the worst. It has been said that if all the skeletons of vessels lying upon or imbedded in the sand between Sandy Hook and Barnegat could be ranged in line, the ghastly array would reach from one point to the other."

The heart of the lighthouse was the lamp and lens. Virtually everything else was simply a tower to support the light, buildings for supplies, and housing for the lighthouse keepers.

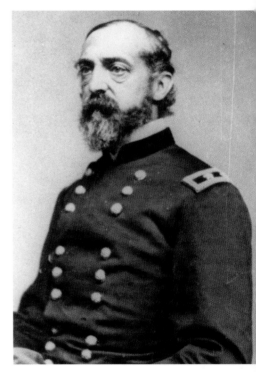

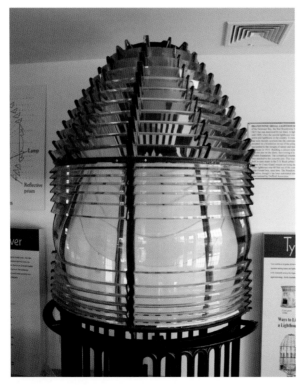

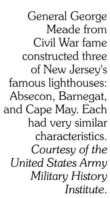

General George Meade from Civil War fame constructed three of New Jersey's famous lighthouses: Absecon, Barnegat, and Cape May. Each had very similar characteristics. *Courtesy of the United States Army Military History Institute.*

The design of the lens was ingenious. Augustin Fresnel, a French physicist and engineer, perfected the system in 1822. So efficient was his design, it captured all but seventeen percent of available light—something never done before. His system of bending and refracting light is still in use today. The lenses came in sizes, known as orders. This is a Fourth Order Lens on exhibit at Tuckerton Seaport.

Lighthouses along the NJ Coast

The lighthouses are listed going from north to south and includes their size (1=largest; 6=smallest), original construction date, and present construction. *(In a few cases there might be only one date if the original and present construction dates are the same)*:

~ Sandy Hook: 3, 1764
~ Twin Lights of the Navesink: 6, 1828, 1862
~ Sea Girt: 4, 1896
~ Barnegat: (formerly) 1, 1835, 1857
~ Hereford Inlet: 4, 1874 (moved in 1913)
~ Absecon: 1, 1856
~ Cape May: 36" radial, 1823, 1859

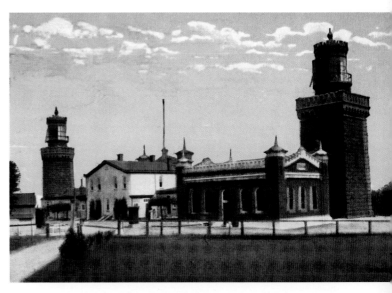

Certainly one of the most architecturally unique lighthouses in the United States, Twin Lights of the Navesink, oversees Sandy Hook Bay and the entrance to New York. Constructed in 1862, it was the first to house a Fresnel lens. In 1898 the light was electrified yielding 25 million candlepower and was the most powerful beacon in the United States and could be seen at a distance of seventy miles.

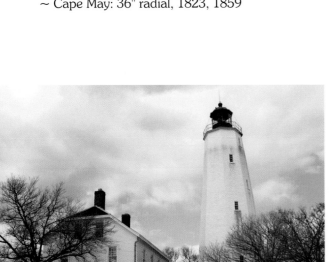

In an effort to forestall dangers of running ashore, a series of lighthouses were constructed along the New Jersey Coast, serving as aids to navigation. They of course serve the primary purpose of preventing ships from crashing ashore. The 103-foot Sandy Hook Lighthouse is the oldest continuously operating lighthouse in America, dating back to 1764. Its beacon can be seen nineteen miles at sea.

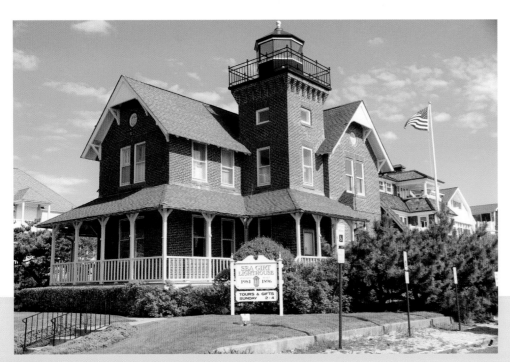

Despite the warnings given to sailors by the lighthouses, they weren't enough to forestall what seemed to be an endless series of tragedies off the New Jersey Coast. One estimate places the number of wrecks off the Jersey Shore at 5,000. Driven ashore by unfavorable winds, usually those blowing from the northeast, early captains were at the mercy of the sea and wind, unable to control their ships. They were blown ashore and wrecked in the heavy surf. Sea Girt Lighthouse, constructed in 1896 lies opposite lifeguard headquarters.

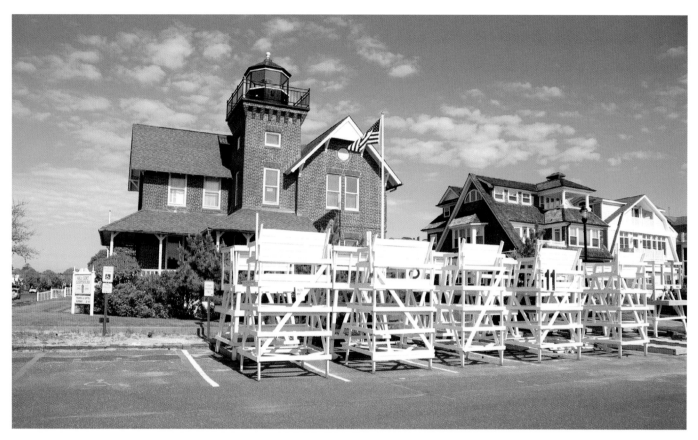

Two eras of lifesaving are represented here in Sea Girt as modern lifeguard stands await the busy summer season outside the nineteenth century lighthouse.

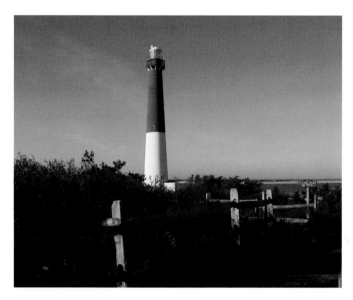

Each lighthouse along the Jersey Coast was distinctively shaped or painted so it could be identified during the day. The unique configuration of each lighthouse throughout the United States was known as a "daymarker." The Barnegat Lighthouse was constructed in 1858 under the direction of George Meade. Located at the northern tip of Long Beach Island, the 172-foot spire is one of the most famous in the United States.

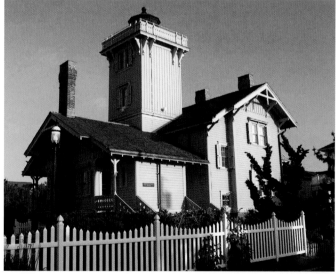

The combination of the distinctive tower architecture, the supply and storage buildings, and the living quarters for the keeper and his assistants gave each lighthouse a distinctive look and character. In some circumstances, the tower was built directly into the living quarters, such as the 1874 Hereford Light in North Wildwood. It housed a fourth order Fresnel lens and was visible thirteen miles at sea.

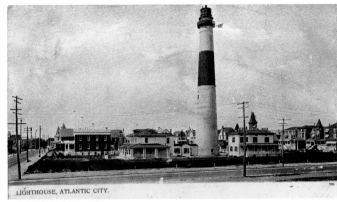

LIGHTHOUSE, ATLANTIC CITY.

Absecon Lighthouse in Atlantic City was the first of three constructed by General George Meade. The 171-foot lighthouse, constructed in 1856, housed a first order Fresnel lens. Seen in the background a bit to the right with the tall peaked roof is the Atlantic City Life-Saving Station.

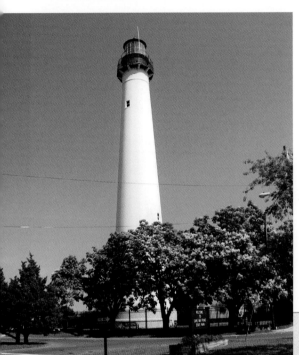

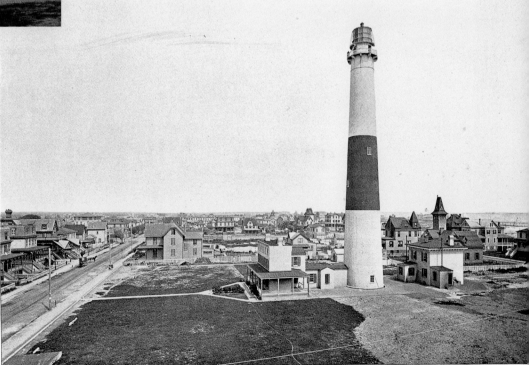

The recently replicated lighthouse keeper's residence at Absecon Light is a museum and tribute to early days of warning ships at sea. At one time, it was right near the ocean but due to land reclamation and construction, now lies several blocks inland. It is open for tours.

Cape May Lighthouse was the third of its type constructed by General George Meade. At 157 feet tall, it still illuminates today, maintained by the State of New Jersey. Constructed in 1859, it is the second oldest continuously operating lighthouse in America.

A rare view of the Absecon Lighthouse again showing the Lifesaving Station to the right of the tower. The lighthouse had a first order Fresnel lens and the beacon could be seen for many miles at sea. The keeper's quarters to the left of the base have been restored. *Courtesy of the Atlantic City Library, Heston Collection.*

ABSECON LIGHTHOUSE

Birth of the United States Life-Saving Service

Lighthouses did not save lives, but instead were used to aid navigation. Yet more needed to be done to prevent the tragic loss of life. The concept of rescue and saving lives was soon to be. The Life-Saving Service's heritage is rooted in the Massachusetts Humane Society. The organization began in 1787 with the construction of small huts or "Humane Houses" along the Massachusetts coastline. They were designed to accommodate shipwrecked sailors with food and shelter but were unattended and subject to theft and vandalism. They did not have lifesaving equipment such as boats to help others who were stranded. The first lifesaving station in America was on Lovell's Island, near Boston.

Eventually lifeboats were added. In 1807, the first surfboat station at Cohassset, near Boston, was completed. Despite an excellent record of lifesaving, all efforts to date had been in just one state — Massachusetts.

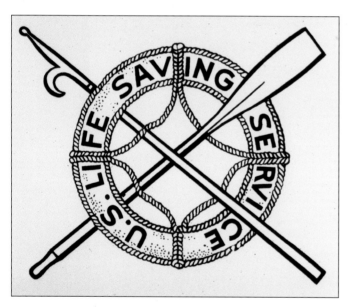

The United States Life-Saving Service was established after shipwrecks close to shore caused thousands of lives to be lost that could have been rescued.

U.S. Life-Saving Service Comes to New Jersey

Based on the successes in Massachusetts, the United States government was petitioned to become involved. The primary advocate was Dr. William A. Newell, who was vacationing with his family at an ironically named hotel — the Mansion of Health — when he witnessed a tragedy. During the evening of August 13, 1839, the northeast winds were blowing hard and steady. The rain beat against the hotel in sheets, and the heavy surf gave

notice to sailors — keep offshore until it blows over. The Austrian brig *Terasto* could no longer fight the wind and surf and was driven ashore three hundred yards offshore as Dr. Newell and other spectators stood by helplessly. There were no survivors, as fourteen men were swept to their deaths that night.

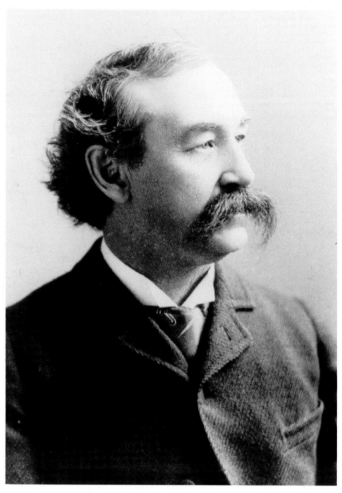

The Life-Saving Service, under Douglass Ottinger, limped along successfully for twenty-two years. Sumner I. Kimball (pictured) would begin the second era of life-saving by taking over and substantially upgrading the Service. Drafted from the Revenue Marine Service, he was appointed General Superintendent of the Life-Saving Service in 1877. Strict, professional, and a real leader, he transformed a relatively loose organization into a highly disciplined, well trained group of professional rescuers with sweeping improvements throughout the organization. *Courtesy of the United States Coast Guard.*

Just three hundred yards of surf separated the men from their foundering ship and the beach. If there was only a way to reach them with a line or boat, perhaps they could have been saved. Dr. Newell was motivated to find the answer ... especially since his home in Manahawkin was right next to the cemetery where those fourteen men were buried.

Dr. Newell not only practiced medicine, but he also pursued a political career. His election to the House of

Representatives afforded him the clout to propose and get approval for a government-sponsored lifesaving service. It was 1848, and the ships kept piling up on shore. Since the time that young William had witnessed the Terasto disaster, 338 ships had been stricken. His colleagues needed little convincing and, in the following year, 1849, the first eight lifeboat stations in the United States were in place — along the Jersey Shore. The original bill provided for surfboats, lifeboats, rockets, carronades (short, light cannon of large caliber, used for short distances), and other rescue apparatus.

The service was established under the auspices of the Revenue Marine, which placed Captain Douglass Ottinger in charge of setting up the stations and equipment along the Jersey Shore. Lifesaving efforts were now clearly established, funded by the United States government. The original eight Surf Boat Stations were:

- ~ Sandy Hook at Spermacetti Cove
- ~ Long Branch at Monmouth Beach
- ~ Deal Beach at Deal
- ~ Shark River at Spring Lake
- ~ Squan Beach at Chadwick's *(a fishing village on Barnegat)*
- ~ Six Mile Beach at Island Beach
- ~ Barnegat at Harvey Cedars
- ~ Long Beach at Beach Haven

Basic Rescue Equipment

Coston Flare: Used for signaling
Beach Apparatus Cart: Used to transport rescue equipment along the beach to a wreck site
Lines: There are three main kinds used; the shot, the whip, and the hawser

 *Shot Line: Using a Lyle Gun, the line is fired to a stricken ship.
 *Whip Line: Used to pull the Lifecar or breeches buoy along the hawser.
 *Hawser: Main support line of the Lifecar or breeches buoys pulled out via a shot line.

Setup: Crotch poles and sand wedges (anchors) to support highly tensioned hawser
Faking Box: Held the shot line in a pattern to prevent fouling
Francis Lifecar: Watertight metal boat that could transport three to five victims to shore
Breeches Buoy: Ring buoy and canvas breeches used to transport a single victim to shore
Boats: The main type of boats used in the beginning were the English Lifeboat and the Beebe/McClellan Surfboat
 *English Lifeboat: Self-bailing, self-righting surfboat rowed to stricken ship
 *Beebe/McClellan Surfboat: Self-bailing, but not self-righting; seaworthy boat rowed to stricken ships; smaller/lighter than English Lifeboat

Other miscellaneous equipment included shovels, spare lines, gunpowder, flares, and a tally board.

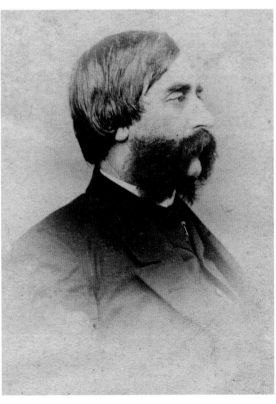

Founder of the United States Life-Saving Service, Dr. William A. Newell called for the establishment of eight stations, which were in place in 1849.

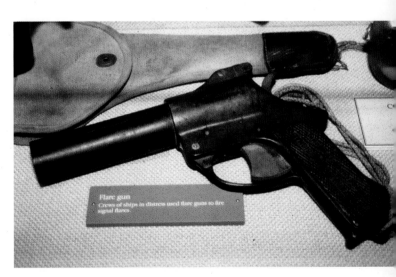

The Coston Gun would fire a flare from the stricken ship to signal shore based rescuers. The Life-Saving Service would respond opposite the ship and attempt to fire a shot line through the rigging. *Courtesy of Sandy Hook Museum.*

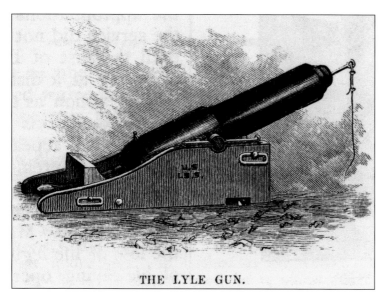

THE LYLE GUN.

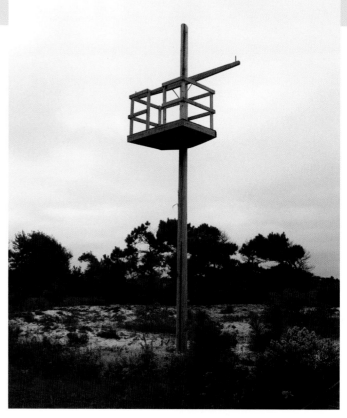

Lines were first shot from shore to the stricken ship. The cannon, developed by David Lyle fired a fourteen pound projectile approximately four hundred yards with an attached "shot line." Their goal was to snag the rigging of the ship. Once the line was retrieved, they pulled a heavier hawser line on board to begin the rescue process.

The boat pole provided a target for land based practice.

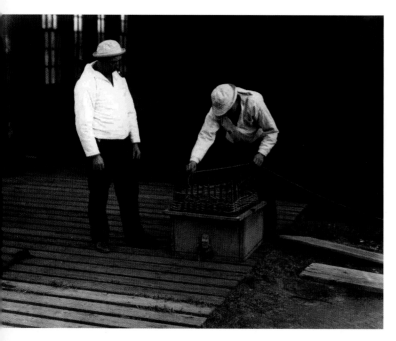

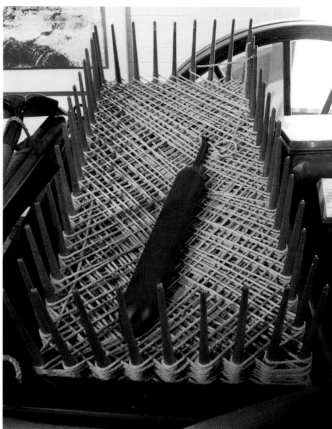

The shot line was fired from a "faking box," a special design that lessened the possibility of the line snarling as it was carried to the ship by the Lyle Gun projectile. The line had to be methodically wrapped in a pattern around the pegs. *Courtesy of NPS/Gateway NRA.*

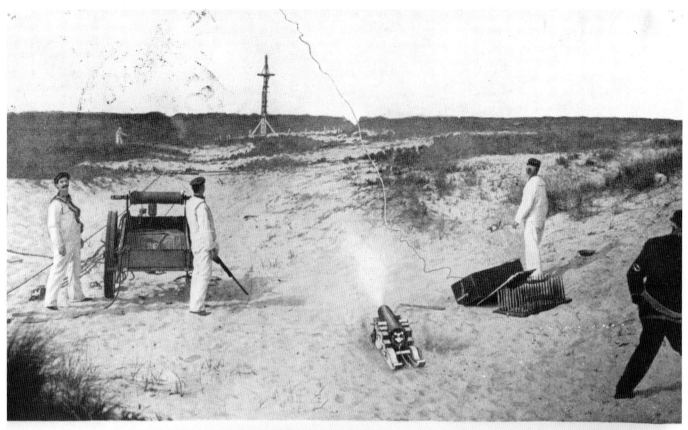

THE LIFE SAVING CREW. SHOOTING THE LIFELINE.

ILLUST. POST CARD CO.,

Land drill attempting to place the shot line over the practice rigging known as a "boat pole." *Courtesy of Sandy Hook archives.*

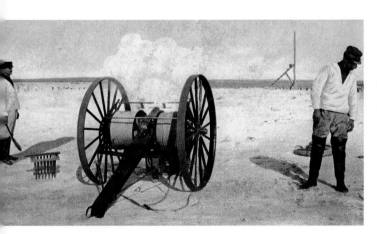

The Life-Saving Service practiced regularly to hone their skill in reaching ships in distress. Crews took great pride in their professionalism fostering a healthy rivalry among stations.

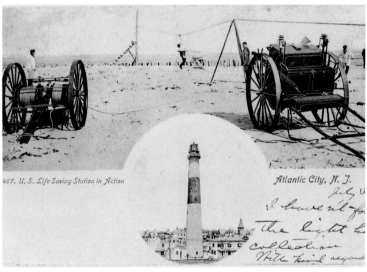

467. U. S. Life Saving Station in Action

Atlantic City, N. J.

Atlantic City Life-Saving Station conducting drills on the beach. Shown are the "beach apparatus" cart and a man in a breeches buoy riding on the line supported by "crotch poles."
Courtesy of the Atlantic City Library, Heston Collection.

The Francis Lifecar

There is debate about who developed the surfcar, a rescue device designed to transport victims from a stricken ship to shore. Was it Douglass Ottinger, first leader of the Life-Saving Service, or Joseph Francis, for whom the device is named? The debate still exists to this date, but Sumner I. Kimball, in later years credited Francis for the invention.

The Lifecar concept worked well for years, but by the 1890s, it began to lose popularity as other technologies developed. Even though the Lifecar worked very well, it was heavy work for the rescuers and a harrowing ride for the victims. By 1899, the Francis Lifecar was rarely, if ever used, replaced by the breeches buoy. Described as a pair of canvas briefs sewn to a circular life preserver suspended by ropes so the victim could sit upright, the breeches buoy improved efficiency.

Joseph Francis developed a rescue vessel in 1849 called the Francis Lifecar. The Lifecar was a 225-pound watertight rescue boat constructed from galvanized metal that held enough air for four to six people for about fifteen minutes. It could not be rowed, paddled nor sailed. It had only one method of propulsion — being pulled along by the whip line.

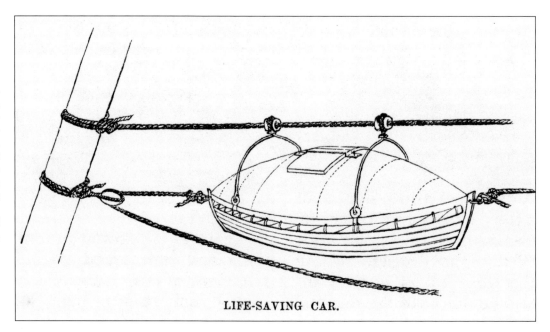

LIFE-SAVING CAR.

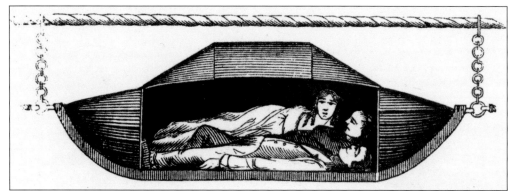

Imagine the terror as victims rode in complete darkness through hurricane surf as they were pulled to shore. Typically the car could carry three to five victims.

The job was simple in concept. Tie a rope between the stricken ship and the shore, and pull people to safety. How this happened in reality was a different story, and one that depends on specialized equipment of the Life-Saving Service.

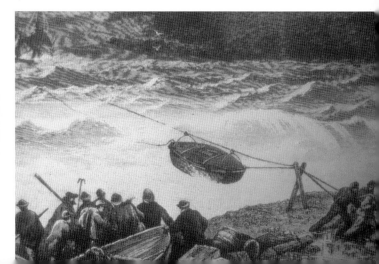

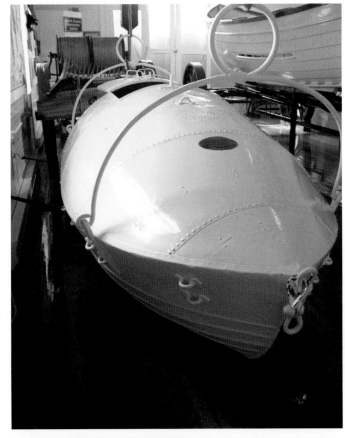

The little double ended airtight skiff had a great debut. In January 1850, just five months after the formation of the Life-Saving Service, the Lifecar rescued two hundred passengers from the British emigrant ship *Ayrshire*, which went aground off the Squan Beach Life-Saving Station. Unfortunately, there were 201 people on board. One man refused to ride inside the tiny craft — he wanted to hold on to the outside. Swept away by the heavy surf, he was the only fatality. The Francis Lifecar rode on the hawser line strung through the rings and pulled by the whip line attached to the bow and stern hooks. Note the watertight hatches on the deck.

traveled long distances. There were constant drills and rivalries between stations.

They established a great record — all totaled throughout the United States, the service saved the lives of 177,286 between 1871 and 1914.

Merger with the Revenue Marine Service

The civilian Life-Saving Service had done its job well. The upstart volunteers begun by Dr. Newell had evolved into a highly-organized, well-disciplined rescue service. However it was showing its age. Men had stayed on long past their prime, and the service became a twelve-month occupation, making it less attractive for younger men.

There were far fewer shipwrecks now, and by the turn of the century the role of the Life-Saving Service began to diminish. Advances in navigation made ocean travel safer. Ships were larger and with powerful engines instead of sails, they could face directly into nor'easters, keeping offshore and away from deadly shoals and communication made navigation much more reliable. They could radio for help when needed, not having to rely on spotters seeing a flare. Shore based stations could be informed exactly what the problem was.

The tie in with the military Revenue Marine Service was logical. It too had run its course and was ripe for reorganization. The end came in 1915. The U.S. Life-Saving Service merged with the Revenue Marine Service to become the United States Coast Guard.

The Second Era: Sumner I. Kimball

Although Dr. Newell introduced the legislation for the Life-Saving Service, it was Captain Douglass Ottinger who actually established the service. It managed to function for twenty-two years organized as volunteers with a paid keeper. They had trouble keeping equipment maintained and upgraded. Sumner I. Kimball arrived on the scene in 1871 and reorganized the service, making it one of the best in the world. The men were issued uniforms and held regular training. As a result, many people held them in high regard for their courage and heroism. Eventually the Life-Saving Service in New Jersey expanded to forty-two locations from Sandy Hook to Cape May, with about three miles distance between each. The service itself spread throughout the United States from coast to coast, including the Great Lakes region.

Men were kept on duty from September 1st to May 1st at $40 a month and the keeper received $60 a month. There were six man crews, one for each oar, and an additional man was put on December 1st. Crews maintained constant patrols in cold weather through soft sand, and

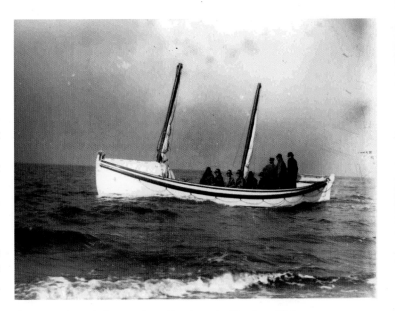

Crews preferred the sturdy self-righting/self-bailing lifeboat. Here, at least the crew was assured the boat would always land upright and be drained of water, but it was a mixed blessing — the boats were extremely heavy and difficult to maneuver. They had to be dragged out onto the beach by horse-drawn carts. *Courtesy of Dorn's Classic Images.*

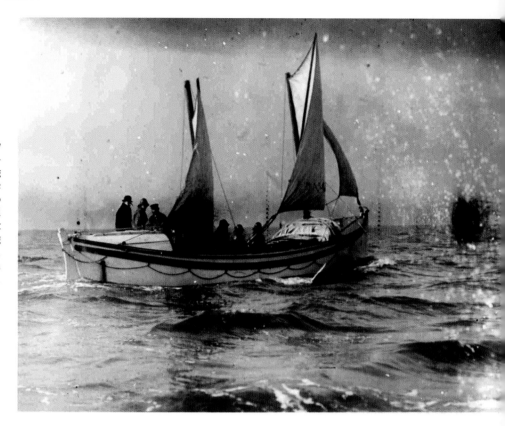

Boats of course, were the mainstay of the Life-Saving Service. Two basic varieties evolved, each serving a different purpose. Pictured here is the English Lifeboat, a 29- to 34-foot, 4,000-pound double end boat that could be rowed by eight men or sailed. It was self-righting — if it capsized, it would right itself; and self bailing — any water taken over the rails would quickly empty. *Courtesy of Dorn's Classic Images.*

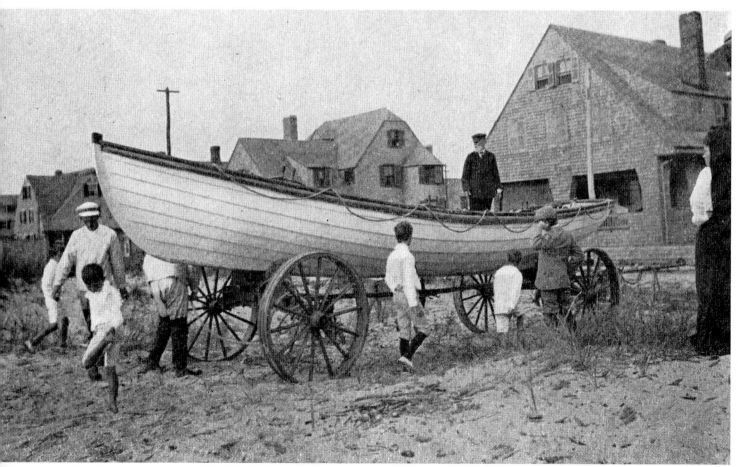

Although the English Lifeboat would go on to become the basis for motorized lifeboats, they were largely replaced by the much lighter and more maneuverable Beebe/McClellan skiff. It was modeled after the time-tested and extremely seaworthy Sea Bright Skiffs. They were good boats and excellent for rescue work. Much easier to launch from the beach into surf, they were 26 1/2 feet long with a 6 1/2-foot beam. Best of all, they could be rowed by six men.

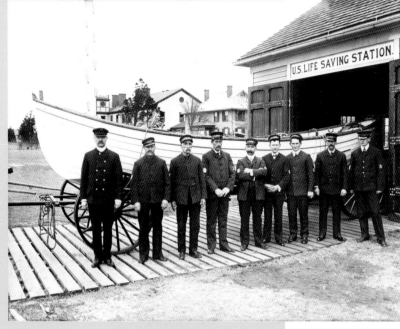

A United States Life-Saving Service crew at Sandy Hook. *Courtesy of Moss Collection, NPS/Gateway NRA.*

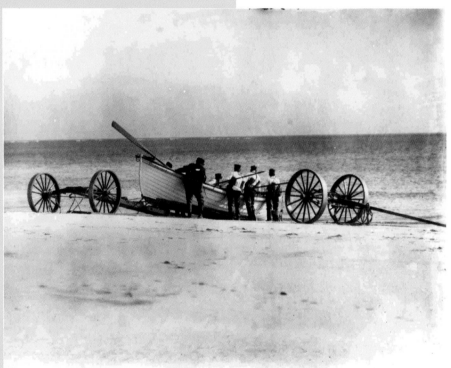

When horses were available, they were used to drag the boats down to the water's edge via boat dollies. The beach apparatus cart carried all essential emergency equipment out on the beach to a site opposite the wreck. The crew at Sea Bright is pictured here with their cart. *Courtesy of Dorn's Classic Images.*

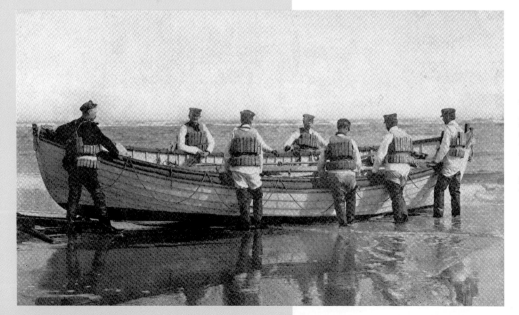

The Atlantic City Life-Saving Crew prepares to launch their double end surfboat. It was approximately twenty-six feet long and was self-bailing, meaning that water taken in would quickly drain from the hull. Note the cork life vests.

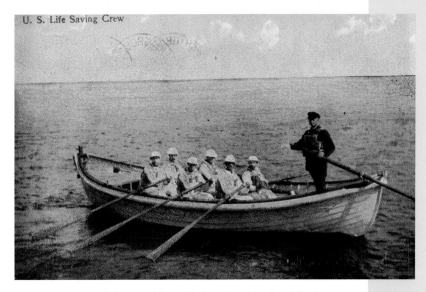

If boats overturned, they could quickly be righted by the skilled crew. In one demonstration at the St. Louis Exposition, the crew, seated at the oars, capsized the craft, righted it, and returned to a rowing position in thirteen seconds.

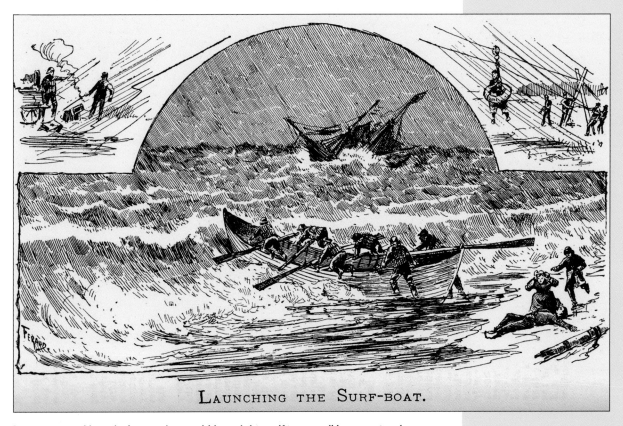

LAUNCHING THE SURF-BOAT.

It was a special breed of man who would launch himself in a small boat against huge surf with driving and sweeping waves, on a bitterly freezing and stormy day in January. Kimball believed in training — constant training. There were weekly drills. Each man had a specific job to do, and it was amazing how quickly they could set up the equipment, fire a line over the drill pole, and affect a practice rescue. There were constant drills and rivalries between stations.

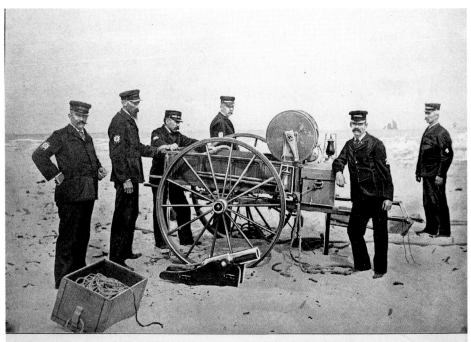

Arriving opposite the wreck, the well drilled crew sprung into action. Each man had specific tasks, and very little needed to be said. It was remarkable how quickly the entire stage could be set in preparation for rescue — usually in under five minutes. This included setting up the Lyle Gun, positioning the faking box holding the shot line, placing the charge and projectile within the gun, digging in sand wedges, erecting the crotch poles, and securing the block and tackle. The gun was aimed, the crew cleared back to a safe distance, and if all went well, the shot line would land across the ship. The crew at Deal Beach in Monmouth County proudly shows their beach apparatus cart which transported the equipment to the wreck site. *Courtesy of Don Stine.*

LIFE-SAVING CREW AND APPARATUS, DEAL BEACH.

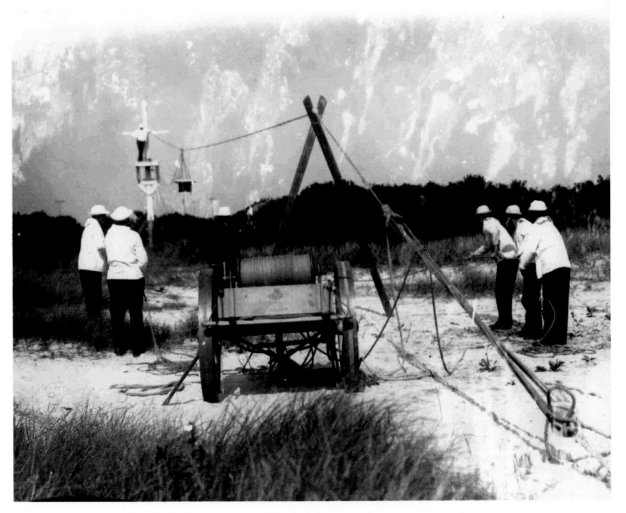

By the turn of the century, the breeches buoy was found to be more effective than the Francis Lifecar. Although it was only possible to rescue one victim at a time, it was felt to be far safer and more efficient than pulling the 225-pound surfcar. *From the Sandy Hook Archives.*

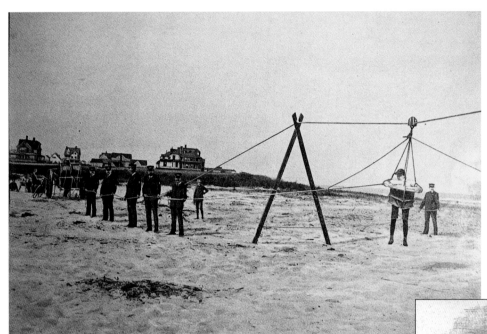

LIFE-SAVING CREW AND BREECHES BUOY, DEAL BEACH.

The Francis Lifecar was abandoned in later years in favor of the breeches buoy. Here, the Deal Beach crew in Monmouth County practices their skills. *Courtesy of Don Stine.*

Eight Surfboat stations were established in 1849. These early 16- x 29-foot stations housed the rescue equipment. Unfortunately, they were often vandalized and had equipment stolen. Crews responded much as a volunteer fire department would today.

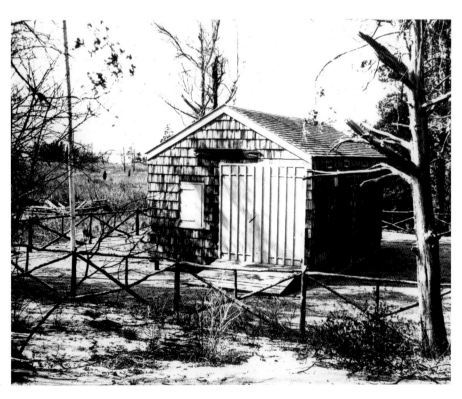

The original surfboat station at Sandy Hook was in place by 1849. *Courtesy of National Archives Collection, NPS/Gateway NRA.*

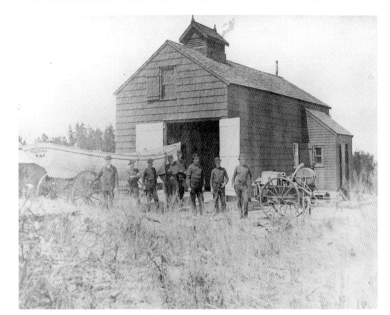

As time progressed through the nine-teenth century, the stations increased in number and architectural sophistication. This is the 1872 Red House Type station at Sandy Hook.
Courtesy NPS/Gateway NRA.

This 1855 life-saving station at Lake Taka-nassee guarded the Long Branch and Elberon beaches. In later years, this station became a pri-vate residence that preservationists now want to turn into a life-saving museum.

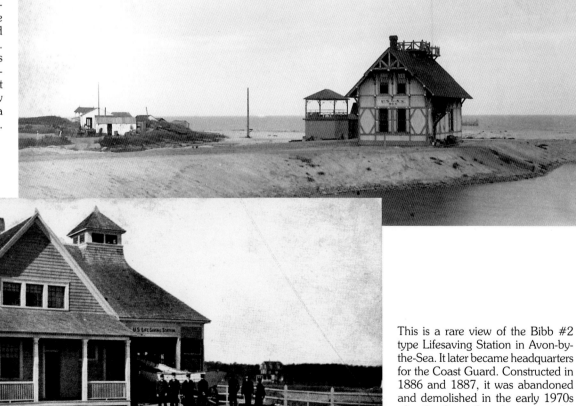

This is a rare view of the Bibb #2 type Lifesaving Station in Avon-by-the-Sea. It later became headquarters for the Coast Guard. Constructed in 1886 and 1887, it was abandoned and demolished in the early 1970s after the Coast Guard constructed a more modern headquarters along the Shark River Inlet.

Published by C. D. Snyder, Real Estate.

U. S. L. S. S. No. 7. Avon by the Sea, N. J

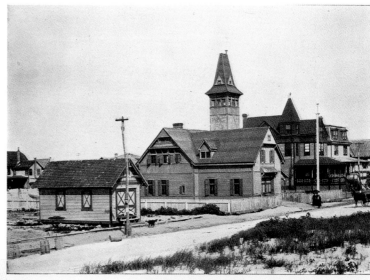

U.S. LIFE SAVING STATION

Architecture of the Atlantic City Life-saving Station was one of only three in New Jersey designed by Paul Pelz. Its design gave comfortable lodging to the crew as well as providing adequate storage of all the rescue gear. *Courtesy of the Atlantic City Library, Heston Collection.*

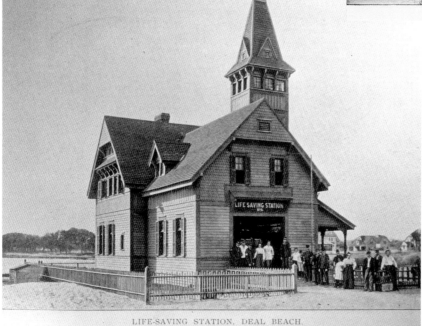

LIFE-SAVING STATION, DEAL BEACH.

Crews were housed in life-saving stations such as this one in Deal Beach in Monmouth County. This beautiful Queen Anne architecture station, built in 1882, was designed by Paul Pelz, who also designed the Library of Congress. The station was opposite Deal Lake at the north end of Asbury Park. *Courtesy of Don Stine.*

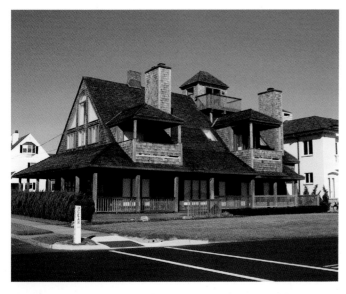

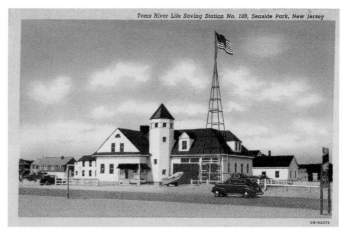

The Spring Lake Life-Saving Station is now a private residence along Ocean Avenue. Constructed in 1896, it was recently featured on "Home & Garden TV." Exclusively appointed, this beautiful home retains the basic design of the original station.

The Toms River Life-Saving Station was one of eleven Jersey Pattern quarters constructed in the mid to late 1890s. The station, constructed in 1899 and located in Seaside Park, was used by the Life-Saving Service for sixteen years before being taken over by the Coast Guard.

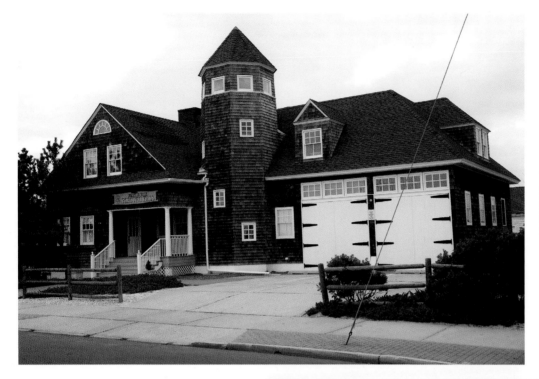

The same station today is used as the Borough Hall in Seaside Park. It is one of several old life-saving stations retro-fitted for modern use.

Ship Bottom Life-Saving Station is another Jersey Pattern station constructed in 1898. International signal flags fly from the radio mast.

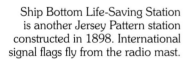

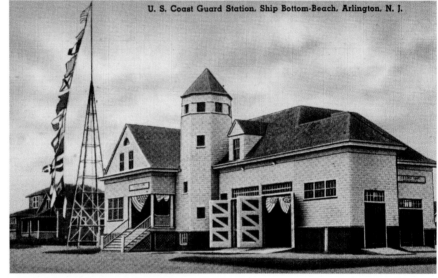

U. S. Coast Guard Station, Ship Bottom-Beach, Arlington, N. J.

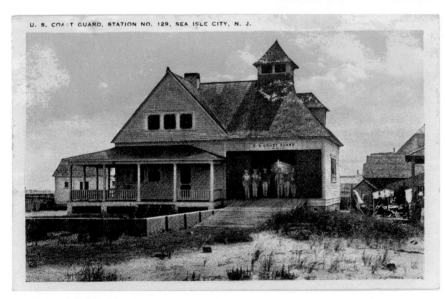

U. S. COAST GUARD, STATION NO. 129, SEA ISLE CITY, N. J.

The Sea Isle City Life-Saving Station was a Bibb #2 style station and was constructed in 1888.

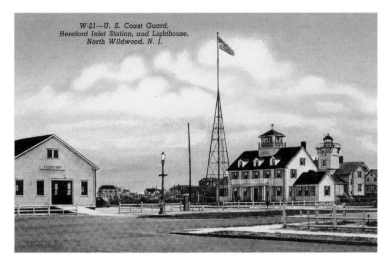

The Hereford Inlet Station is a more modern type and located in North Wildwood. It replaced the original station built in 1888.

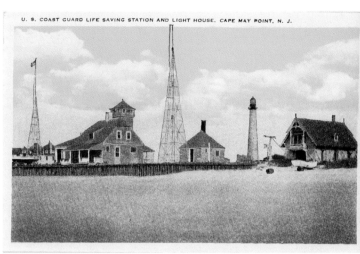

The life-saving station and lighthouse at Cape May Point: note the two architectural styles — the Duluth Style between the signal towers and the 1876 type to the right. Built for the 1876 Philadelphia Centennial Exposition, it then moved to Cape May.

Dragged Over the Top of the Jetty

Michael "Spike" Fowler,
Lifeguard Supervisor
Monmouth County Park System

Although I've seen thousands of rescues over the years, one of the hairiest was at Seven Presidents Oceanfront Park in Long Branch. We had "red flag" conditions at our park, which is part of our preventive lifeguarding protocol: if the water is too rough, don't let them in! Our job was to "keep people out of the water!" I was at the Atlantic Avenue beach with Laura Jean Fronapfel and several other guards. Just to the north of our property is a "private beach," as we called it; it was adjacent to our park, but not in our jurisdiction.

Some foolish person decided to ignore our warnings and swim outside our area. We could see the beach and see him and we knew he could see our red flag. He was several hundred yards north of Park System property. We had already whistled out several bathers before him. We did this as a "courtesy" to warn people and protect them from their own lack of judgment.

Despite our frantic whistle blowing, this middle-aged, foolhardy man, unbelievably, was swimming right into the mouth of a horrendous rip current and we realized immediately

this was going to be a problem. We grabbed the line bucket, several rescue cans and sprinted up north, off our property. Laura Jean, a college scholarship swimmer had already hooked up to the rescue flotation device and rescue line. We arrived on scene, right alongside a jetty and she entered the water along with another rescuer with a free RFD (not connected to the rescue line). By now the victim was swept quite a distance off shore, far beyond the breakers. I was feeding the line and would be the "line puller." Several other guards had arrived on scene as well. Just as Laura Jean had positioned the victim on the rescue device and signaled us to start pulling, a large wave swept them north, and the line was now over the jetty and the only alternative was keep on pulling. Well, they were dragged over the top of the jetty rocks, but luckily another wave had "cushioned" the blow somewhat. Everyone made it safely to shore — the victim had escaped any injury and Laura Jean just had some minor scrapes and bruises.

Although it wasn't professional, I delivered an excoriating and lengthy treatise on the victim's lack of judgment, highlighting his stupidity and how he had placed my crew at peril. He slinked away ashamed and embarrassed and actually I felt pretty good about it. "This will teach him a lesson he won't soon forget," I thought to myself.

Laura Jean was the heroine of the day and it was one of the more exciting rescues I've taken part in. She was one of my best rescuers. That day for certain, I knew we had made a difference. I still shudder when I think of what could have happened.

Chapter Three

Lifeguarding in the Early Days

As the hot summer months fell upon the urban and farm population, it was fashionable to head "down the shore." Frolicking freely in the surf brought great delight for young and old alike. After all, what could happen on a beautiful summer's day? The ocean brought fun and relief from the heat, dust and insects.

Safety at the beach was an important issue during the mid-nineteenth century. The number of bathers losing their lives each summer to the call of the surf motivated the early hotel owners to take precautions. An 1874 pamphlet, *Long Branch and Its Environs: A Full Description of "The Summer Capitol" and the Surrounding Country*, contained two advertisements from hotels. The Howland Hotel stated "competent bathers always on duty" while the Central Hotel, using a slight modification, read "competent bathers always on hand." It was also good marketing! They could advertise that their beaches were free from the dangers associated with ocean bathing. Despite warnings, on average, a dozen people lost their lives each year in the Atlantic City surf.

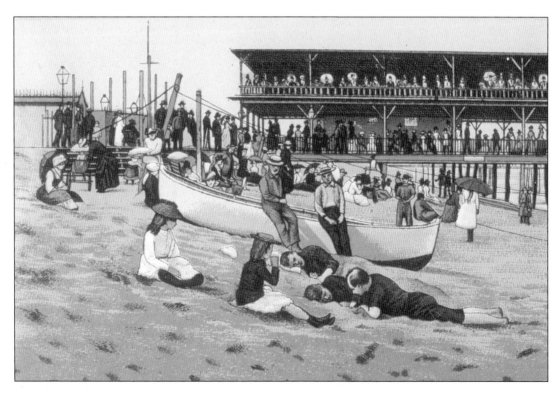

In 1865, Manie Lawlor drowned in the surf off Atlantic City, prompting local hotel proprietors and bathhouse keepers to install bathing lines. They wisely didn't call them bathing lines — they called them "lifelines." These proved insufficient as unwary swimmers went beyond them, resulting in additional drownings. This is an 1890s view in Asbury Park.

One of the first safety innovations was bathing poles supporting lines strung between them. This concept became a New Jersey bathing beach standard for over a century. Ropes didn't rescue anyone struggling in the surf, and once a hapless bather was swept beyond the lines, they were useless.

In 1874, hotels in Long Branch offered guests "competent bathers" as a precursor to lifeguards as seen in a pamphlet titled *Long Branch and Its Environs: A Full Description of "The Summer Capitol" and the Surrounding Country*. Proprietors felt their beach was "unsurpassed upon the Atlantic Coast" and in an odd choice of words "unexceptionable for bathing."

25

HOWLAND'S HOTEL,
Long Branch,
H. HOWLAND & SONS,
Proprietors.

Beach for bathing unsurpassed upon the Atlantic coast; competent bathers always on duty.

Address,

H. HOWLAND & SONS,

LONG BRANCH, N. J.

CENTRAL HOTEL,
Long Branch,
H. C. SHOEMAKER, Proprietor.

This Hotel is newly built, commodious, and well furnished; also completely fitted with all modern improvements, and being situated on the central part of the beach, is most convenient to all other hotels, the depot and Atlantic block.

Open throughout the year.

PRICES REASONABLE.

Beach in front unexceptionable for bathing.

COMPETENT BATHERS ALWAYS ON HAND,

P. O. Address,

H. C. SHOEMAKER,

East Long Branch.

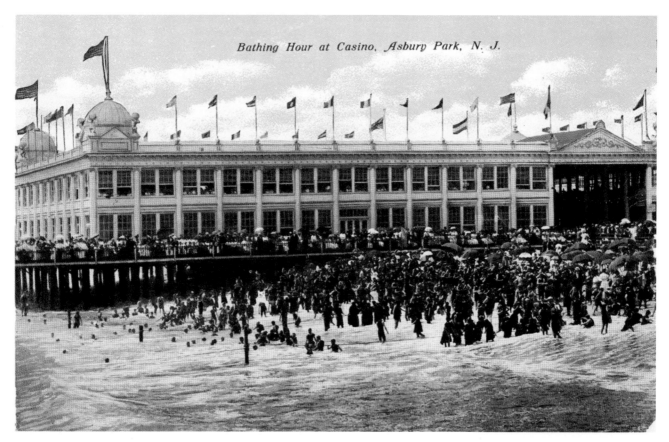

Bathing Hour at Casino, Asbury Park, N. J.

Throngs would gather during the "bathing hour" as illustrated here in Asbury Park.

Captain William Tell Street conceived of a contrivance known as the "bathing car" — a large wired cage with attached floats. Designed for twofold purposes, it could transport the timid into and out of the surf while maintaining modesty standards of the day. People in the latter part of the nineteenth century were fearful of ocean bathing and considered it dangerous. The bathing car could hold approximately a dozen bathers who would reel themselves out and in via a pulley and cable connected to an offshore anchor. The serendipitous benefit, in the day of segregated bathing, was females were able to avoid the eyes of amorous male onlookers.

Despite the seeming security of bathing lines, sometimes people became distressed and needed rescue. Thus was born a new approach to lifesaving, following the traditions that started so many years before.

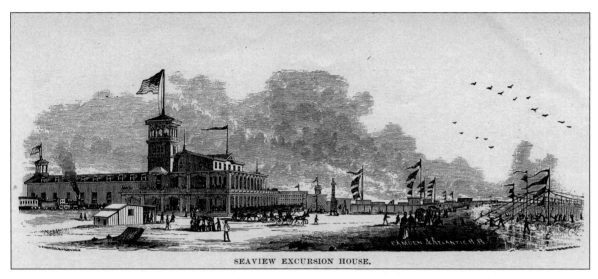

SEAVIEW EXCURSION HOUSE.

Captain William Tell Street's Patented Lifelines for Safety and Amusement consisted of cables strung between poles and anchored offshore with one important modification. Vertical lines were hung every nine feet from the ropes enabling bathers to dangle from them and pass from rope to rope. Apparently it gave great reassurance to bathers, particularly females who preferred the lifelines over the accompaniment of gentlemen. They were first placed on the bathing beaches off the New Excursion Hotel followed by installations at Congress Hall, the Seaview Excursion House and the United States Hotel in Atlantic City. *Alfred M. Heston Collection – Atlantic City Free Public Library.*

Volunteer Lifesavers

There is no date or record establishing when volunteers began plying their trade in Atlantic City, but it was prior to 1855. There is no doubt, however that volunteers were the first lifeguards in New Jersey. Not all enjoyed a positive reputation as it is chronicled that "con-men" would stage fake rescues to generate tips from compassionate beachgoers. The volunteers did not have stations or lifeguard benches. They would simply walk the beaches with a ring buoy, in search of people in danger. Swimming out through the surf, they would drag the victim to shore, towing them on the life preserver. They would then hope for a donation, often passing a hat.

Volunteer Life-Saving Stations, Atlantic City Directory 1882-1883

~ **Bradford Brothers, "The Rescue Life Guard"**: Established 1876, on duty every day and evening, from July 1st to September 30th. Crew — Christopher P. Bradford, Michael G. Bradford, Edward Bradford, John Deane, and George Mullarkey. On the beach between New York Avenue and Indiana Avenue.

~ **Rutter Brothers, "The Volunteer Life Guard"**: On the beach, ocean end of States Avenue. On duty every day and evening, from July 1st to September 30th. Crew — Henry Rutter, Jr. and Samuel Rutter.

On May 18, 1900, Captain Charles E. Clark, a former cowboy, received the Silver Medal of the Volunteer Life Saving Corps of New York. Known colorfully as the "Velvet Coated Hero" referring to his beach costume, the award was presented for the rescue of a drowning boy the previous season. According to the May 19, 1900 *New York Times*, Captain Clark bravely jumped from Young's Ocean Pier, breaking his leg in the process. Despite his injury, he safely landed the boy on the shore, saving his life. In his career as a volunteer lifeguard, he is credited with saving "no fewer than 700 persons," traveling dutifully from beach to beach with his personal ring buoy slung over his shoulder. Captain Clark died in 1918.

Donations received from volunteers could be construed as a windfall, or as the ultimate insult. One day, Henry Rutter of the Rutter Brothers rescued Jacob Whiting, a wealthy Philadelphian. Whiting was so grateful that he "advanced" Henry $500, which Henry used to go into the bathhouse business. The business was so successful that in 1907 he refused an offer of $100,000 for his bathhouse property.

In 1869, Paul Boynton, an expert swimmer, who several years later organized the railroad crews, was one lifeguard who, apparently, took the offer of payment as an insult. When his gentleman victim was dragged ashore after being swept to sea, he offered his rescuer $.50. Paul Boynton quickly returned $.49 quipping he usually did not accept more than a life was worth.

In 1872, Captain Boynton organized the first volunteer lifeguards on the beach in Atlantic City. He was stationed on the beach in front of the Seaview Excursion House. He was paid by the Camden & Atlantic Railroad and by contributions from beach patrons. His diligence resulted in saving many bathers who, no doubt, would have drowned. His success proved the need to expand this service and each year saw more and more guards added to the beach.

The volunteer concept worked better than nothing, but was not ideal. With no work standards or regular pay, volunteers could rarely be counted on to perform their duties. But as the volunteer concept expanded up and down the coast, Atlantic City made strides forward with a new idea — paid beach patrols. The dawn of lifeguarding had come to the Jersey Shore.

The First New Jersey Lifeguards

Ocean lifeguarding developed in several locations concurrently along the New Jersey Shore. It became, in large part, a response to the growth of resorts. While Atlantic City has been widely considered the pioneer of the ocean beach patrol, other shore communities like Asbury Park, Ocean Grove, and Cape May all established their crews much earlier than the majority of municipalities. As resorts sprang up, more and more people took to the sea to experience the refreshing delights that the Atlantic Ocean offered.

The next development in New Jersey lifeguarding was Constables of the Surf assisted by volunteers. According to Frank Butler's *Book of the Boardwalk*, the first constable, William S. Cazier, started in Atlantic City in 1855 when the council appointed two men to safeguard bathers. He was paid $117 for that season of work.

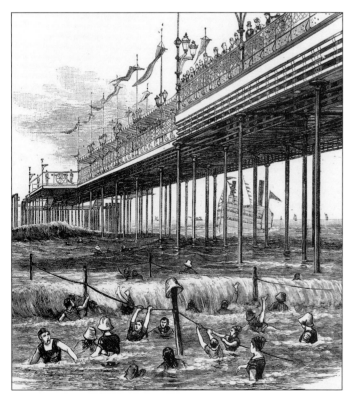

Lifelines for bathing are clearly shown alongside the pier in Long Branch in 1879 in this illustration titled "Bathing in the shade beneath the pier." The steamship *Plymouth Rock* is maneuvering for docking. *Frank Leslie's Illustrated Newspaper, August 23, 1879; courtesy of George H. Moss, Jr.*

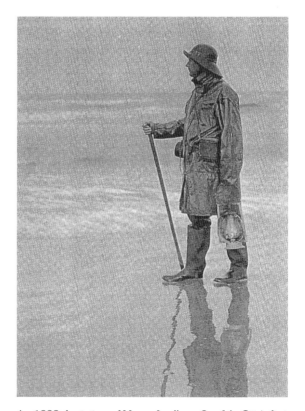

An 1882 depiction of Henry Ludlam, Sea Isle City's first marshal (lifeguard) looking at the sea. He was assigned to patrol the waters' edge four times daily. *Courtesy of Dr. Thomas P. McCann.*

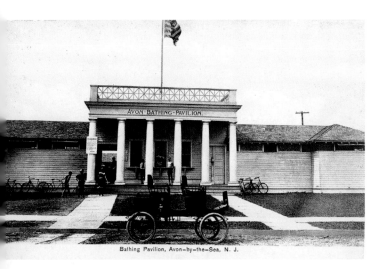

Day trippers would come to swim and change at popular bathhouse facilities such as this 1909 view in Avon-by-the-Sea. The facility housed a swimming pool and lockers. Bathing suits were often rented for the day.

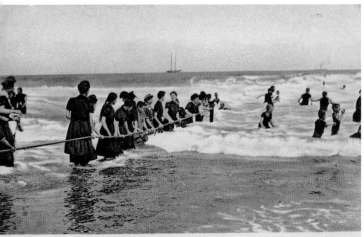

Although Captain Street's system never achieved great popularity, the concept of bathers hanging on to ropes and poles did. This was the modus operandi for early bathers, and there are many postcard views with large numbers of bathers hanging on to ropes. This gave rise to the term "fanny dunking" — holding on to the ropes and dipping one's posterior into the surf.

Rope and pole systems would prevail for at least one hundred years, and they were last seen along the New Jersey Coast in the mid-1960s, when they were replaced with more modern systems of ropes with floats. The early floats were often beer kegs modified with rings with which to attach the ropes. This 1906 view in Bradley Beach shows what seems to be a lifeguard sitting on his rescue reel.

The Atlantic City Council employed additional men in 1875 under the authority of the police department and, by 1884 there were twenty-five Constables of the Surf, making them the oldest operational beach patrol in the United States. After the bathing hours were up, which incidentally was during the hottest part of the day, they changed back into their police uniforms and resumed patrol. However, the guards continued to receive donations from appreciative patrons, a practice long since discontinued.

Would the mere presence of Constables of the Surf scare early beachgoers? Apparently some thought so and wanted to "soften" the idea that surf bathing could be dangerous. An 1877 railroad brochure promoting the nearby resort of Cape May knew well the benefits of public relations.

> Lifelines, as a matter of course are entirely unnecessary and unknown, and the lifeboats, which ride beyond the surf during the hours devoted to bathing, seem to represent a useless precaution. Not withstanding this, the vigilance of their crews while thus hovering outside the multitude disporting in the breakers, presents a sense of security which their watchful care induces, and is at once inviting and reassuring to the weaker or more timid of the bathers in the surf.

City policemen continued this work until the arrival of paid lifeguards on June 12, 1892. Atlantic City continued to grow and with it the beach patrols which protected its citizens and tourists. By the dawn of the twentieth century, the city employed fifty-five lifeguards. This number grew to sixty-four by 1910.

Not counting the volunteers, the technical start of lifeguarding in New Jersey was 1855. Lifeguarding in Ocean Grove followed in 1876. According to the Ocean Grove Campmeeting Association's records, bathing concessions were approved in 1877 in the North End to J. Ross and T.W. Lillagore at the South End. Asbury Park was not far behind in providing rescue services and crews were in place around or slightly prior to 1896.

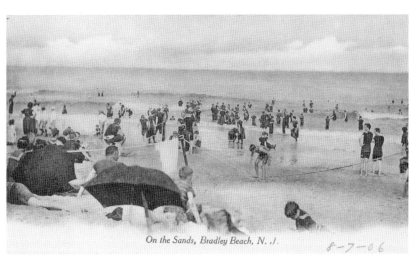

On the Sands, Bradley Beach, N. J.

In Cape May, billed as "America's Oldest Resort," bathing houses hung ropes off the beach in 1845. In later years whaleboats "manned with stout hearts and ready hands" were stationed on beaches during the bathing season. By 1865, the larger hotels hired crews to man surfboats. Rivalries developed among the hotel crews and lifeboat races were held to entertain summer guests.

The popularity of the Jersey Shore and its beaches grew steadily through the latter part of the nineteenth century. Hotel and innkeepers as well as boardwalk and resort proprietors saw great profit potential. Atlantic City and Cape May were booming. Town fathers had to respond to the growing number of bathers and the risks they faced. Fatalities and beach incidents were not good for public relations and bad news in the newspapers could cut revenues. Crews, slowly at first and then much more quickly, emerged to meet the rescue and first aid needs of their patrons.

Jersey Shore Lifeguard Beginnings

~ Cape May Bathhouses: Lifelines, 1845
~ Atlantic City: Volunteers, 1855
~ Atlantic City: Constables of the surf, 1855
~ Atlantic City Hotels: Lifelines, 1865
~ Cape May Bathhouses and Hotels: Paid, 1865
~ Atlantic City: Organized Volunteers, 1872
~ Ocean Grove: Bathing Masters, 1872
~ Long Branch Hotels, Competent Bathers, 1874
~ Ocean Grove, Paid, 1876

~ Sea Isle City, Patrol Marshal, 1882
~ Atlantic City, Paid, 1892
~ Asbury Park, Paid, circa 1896
~ Ocean City, Paid, 1898
~ Ventnor, Paid, 1903
~ Wildwood, Paid, 1905
~ Avalon: Paid & Bathing Masters, 1905
~ Spring Lake, Paid, 1906
~ Holly Beach, Paid, 1907
~ Margate (known as S. Atlantic City), Paid, 1908
~ Seaside Heights, Paid, 1910
~ Cape May, Paid, 1911
~ Stone Harbor, Paid, 1912
~ North Wildwood, Paid, 1914
~ Beach Haven, Paid, 1916
~ Ortley Beach Beach Patrol: Paid, 1917
~ Sea Isle City: One lifeguard, 1917
~ Sea Isle City Beach Patrol: Paid, 1919
~ Wildwood Crest: Paid, 1921
~ Arlington Beach Patrol: Paid, 1926
~ Lavallette: Paid, 1926
~ Ship Bottom: Paid, 1926
~ Avon-by-the-Sea: Paid, 1929
~ Manasquan: Paid, (circa) 1930
~ Mantoloking Beach: Bathing Masters & Watchmen, 1930
~ Harvey Cedars Beach Patrol: Paid, 1932
~ Upper Township: Paid, 1932
~ Belmar: Paid, 1933
~ Long Beach Township: Volunteers, 1933
~ Sea Girt: Paid, 1933
~ Long Beach Township: Paid, 1936
~ Brigantine: Paid, 1938
~ Island Beach State Park Beach Patrol: Paid, 1962
~ Sandy Hook (Gateway N.R.A.): Paid, 1962
~ Monmouth County Park System: Paid, 1977

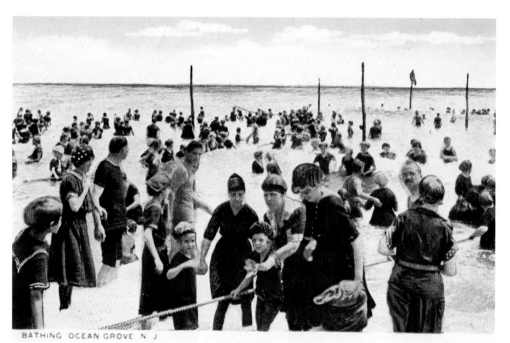

BATHING OCEAN GROVE N J

The poles, aside from being high maintenance also caused quite a few injuries. Bathers knocked into the poles would often emerge from the ocean covered with bruises, or scrapes from the barnacle encrusted poles. Bathers unfortunate enough to ride a wave into the pole were subject to more serious head and neck injuries. If knocked unconscious the risk of being drawn beneath the surface posed a drowning problem.

On June 12, 1892, the Atlantic City Beach Patrol officially was added to the city payroll with their first two paid lifeguards, Jim Jefferies and Nick Headley. Their white belts had a loop in the back to which they would fasten their rescue device. *Alfred M. Heston Collection – Atlantic City Free Public Library.*

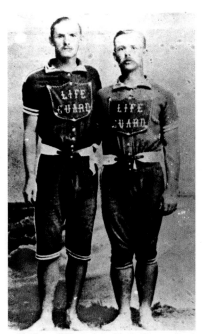

The first paid lifeguards in Atlantic City were Dan Headley and Nick Jefferies, hired in 1892.

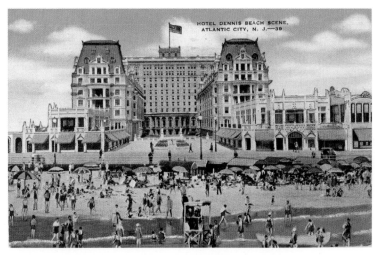

As the Civil War came to an end, Atlantic City emerged as the state's leading resort, paving the way for many to follow. This backwater town quickly became a beautiful city resort sporting a boardwalk that some claimed was the "Promenade of America."

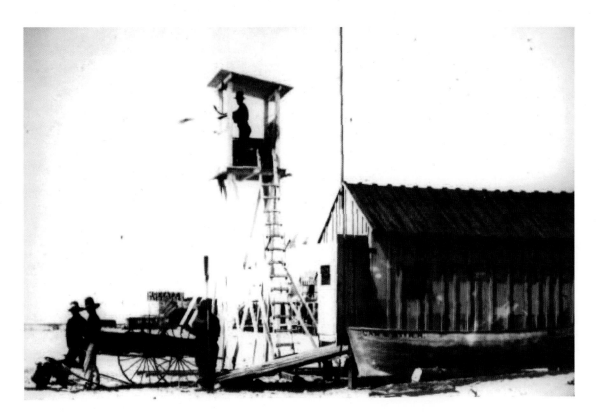

The railroads had a stake in beach safety, so they were the early promoters of lifeguarded beaches. Their bills told of safety at the swimming beaches, the destination of many trains. This rare photo of a high tower was erected by the Camden & Atlantic Railroad to oversee bathers and was perhaps the first lifeguard stand in New Jersey. It could only be reached by a tall ladder. The sign on the building reads "Camden & Atlantic Life Guards." *Courtesy of the Atlantic Heritage Center.*

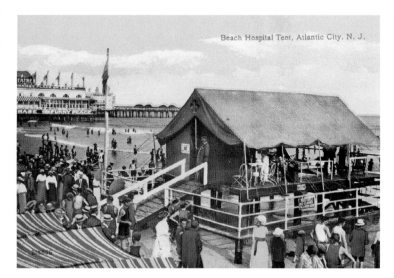

An interesting feature of the beach patrol in Atlantic City was its on-site medical services which started in 1904 with the appointment of Dr. John T. Beckwith as beach surgeon. In the days before rapid response teams capable of whisking accident victims off to hospitals and trauma centers by speedy EMT staffed ambulances or helicopters, on-site medical treatment often meant the difference between life and death. This was provided at "beach hospital tents." According to the Atlantic City Life Guards Beneficial Association, in 1918 six doctors were stationed at the hospital tents and took care of 5,099 cases while the guards made 674 rescues aided by thirty-eight surfboats, fifty can buoys, and two hundred rim buoys.

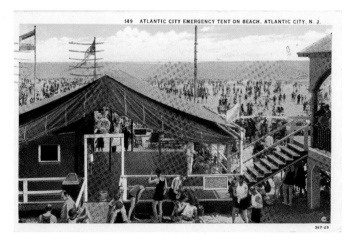

By 1909, things had come a long way. This year saw the creation of the Atlantic City Life Guards' Beneficial Association which was dedicated to providing medical services to the lifeguards and their families, as well as beach patrons. With medical tents right on the beach, doctors were able to respond quickly for everything from splinters and jellyfish stings, to emergency resuscitation.

This early view in Ocean Grove shows bathing poles and a lifeguard stand. Lifeguards had one woolen suit with a red top and black trunks. The president of the Campmeeting Association gave approval for them to be removed "once in a while" in 1937.

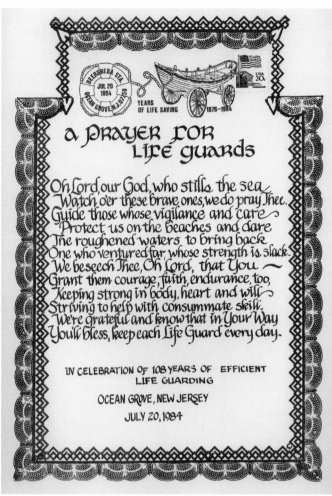

a PRAYER FOR LIFE GUARDS

Oh Lord, our God, who stills the sea
Watch o'er these brave ones, we do pray Thee.
Guide those whose vigilance and care
Protect us on the beaches and dare
The roughened waters, to bring back
One who ventured far, whose strength is slack.
We beseech Thee, Oh Lord, that You —
Grant them courage, faith, endurance, too,
Keeping strong in body, heart and will
Striving to help with consummate skill.
We're grateful and know that in Your Way
You'll bless, keep each Life Guard every day.

IN CELEBRATION OF 108 YEARS OF EFFICIENT LIFE GUARDING

OCEAN GROVE, NEW JERSEY

JULY 20, 1984

By 1872 Ocean Grove had established Bathing Masters. These gentlemen were hired by the local hotels to regulate the bathing of their guests. They determined the bathing hours and whether it was time for men or women to enter the surf. They would also patrol the beaches to check for people in distress. This "Prayer for Life Guards" celebrates 108 years of lifeguarding in 1984, documenting their beginning in 1876.

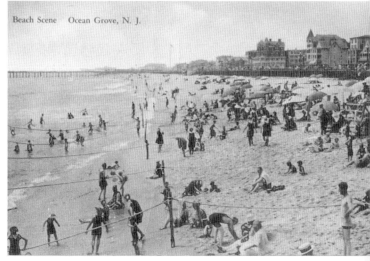

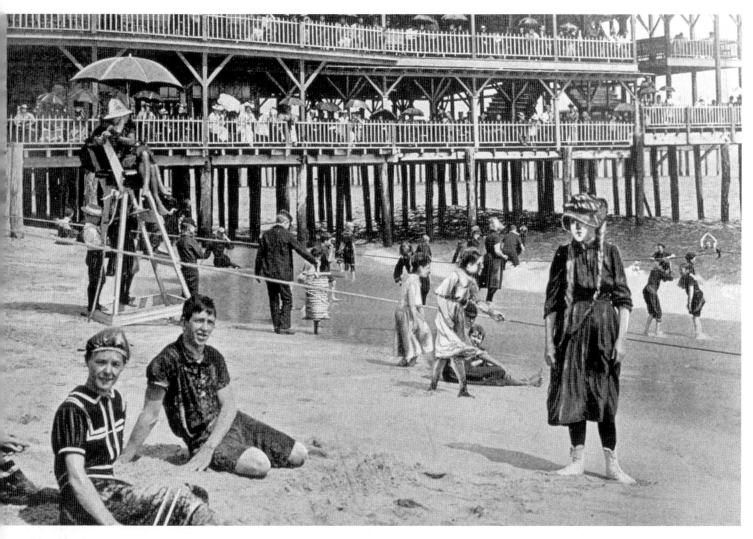

The oldest known picture of Asbury Park Lifeguards shows them in 1896 at the Fourth Avenue Pavilion. *Courtesy of Don Stine.*

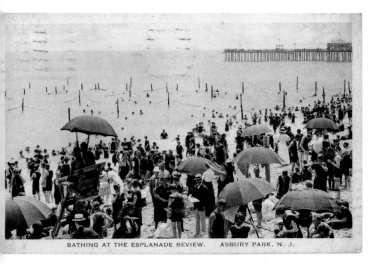

BATHING AT THE ESPLANADE REVIEW. ASBURY PARK, N. J.

Asbury Park grew rapidly as a shore resort and their beaches were packed with tourists on a daily basis. This 1921 photo shows a gentleman with a jacket and bowtie.

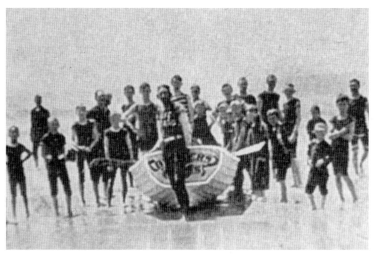

Ocean City's popular volunteer Joseph Krause is shown here in the early 1890s. *Courtesy of Fred Miller.*

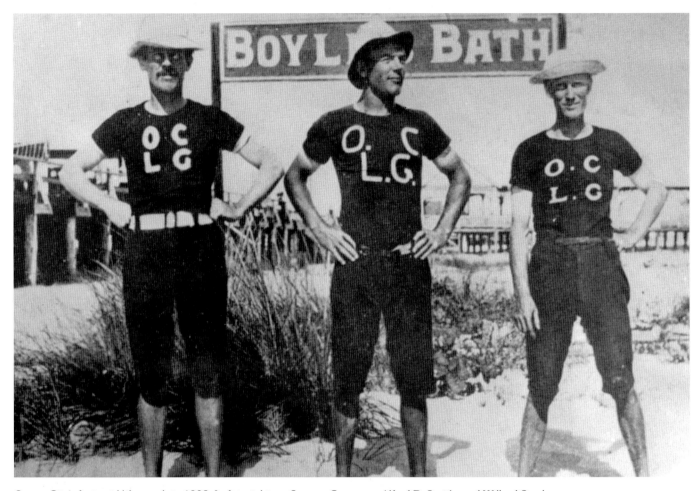

Ocean City's first paid lifeguards in 1902. Left to right are Somers Cameron, Alfred R. Smith, and Willard Steelman. Apparently the lettering was "homemade." *Courtesy of Fred Miller.*

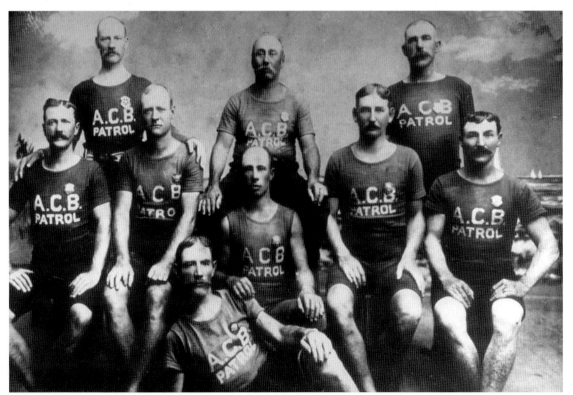

First employed in 1855, Constables of the Surf in Atlantic City would vacate their regular patrol duties daily during the bathing hours — between 11 a.m. and 1:30 p.m., changing into bathing costumes. They would patrol the beaches, complete with their badge pinned to their uniform, and make rescues as necessary. At 1:30, they changed back into their police uniform. By 1884, there were twenty-five constables who worked until 1892 when the City hired their first paid lifeguards. *Alfred M. Heston Collection – Atlantic City Free Public Library.*

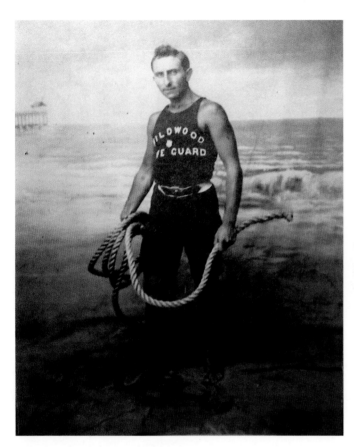

Wildwood Lifeguard circa 1900. *Courtesy of the Wildwood Historical Society.*

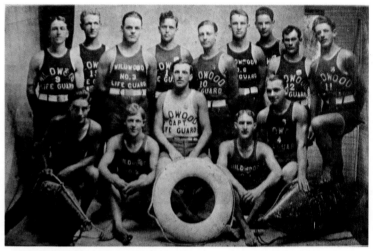

Wildwood Lifeguards in 1914. *Courtesy of the Wildwood Historical Society.*

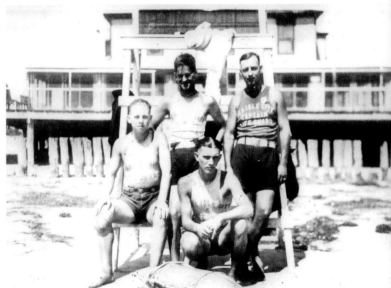

Prior to 1919, Sea Isle City fathers relied on private lifeguards to protect the patrons of the beachfront hotels. Volunteers were always responding to calls for help which happened often along the city's beaches. Captain Coleman worked privately for hotels and volunteers. As his reputation grew, he was asked to start the beach patrol. Pictured front left to right — James Giblin, D.A. Duross; back Thomas Ryan, Captain Jack Coleman. *Courtesy of Dr. Thomas P. McCann.*

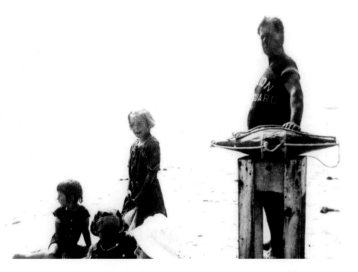

A turn-of-the-century photo of an Avalon lifeguard also shows an early rescue can constructed of metal. *Courtesy of the Avalon Free Public Library.*

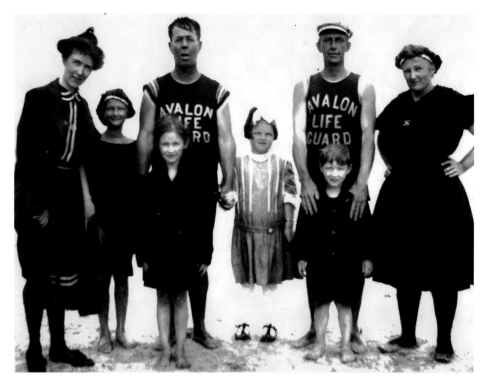

Inaugural Avalon lifeguard crew members, Captain Walter Smith and Lieutenant Howard High pose with family members in this 1905 photo. The beaches were open from 10 a.m. to 4 p.m. during July and August. Lifeguards served as policemen at night. *Courtesy of the Avalon Free Public Library.*

A Standing Ovation

Ted Olsen, Beach Captain
Monmouth County Park System

Toward the end of September, when the ocean usually gets rough, a dramatic rescue occurred at Seven President's Oceanfront Park in Long Branch. We were on patrol when we spotted three teenage boys playing in knee-high water, just north of a massive rip current. One got knocked down and within seconds got swept south toward the mouth of the rip current. One of his friends tried to help but he too lost his balance and began to get swept toward the mouth of the rip. Soon, they were being pulled rapidly offshore in the now massive rip current.

The teens were instantly aware of the situation they were in, and began "doggy paddling" back to shore. This rudimentary style of swimming was no match for this rip current. The third boy, still in shallow water began to frantically call and wave to us. But as soon as he got our attention, he foolishly swam after his friends. Like his friends, he was not a strong swimmer and got swept into the rip current. Just within the blink of eye, three kids who had been playing and laughing in shallow water were now in serious trouble forty yards off shore.

I radioed for assistance, while my lieutenant and rookie entered the water to try and rescue the youngsters. Unfortunately, the radio call was not received and to make matters worse, there were no backup guards nearby.

I instinctively knew time was of the essence and swam into the rip, sprinting to the victims. Once I reached them, two were panicking. They tried climbing over the rescue cans reaching

for the guards in an attempt to save their lives. With one boy I had to squeeze pressure points under his arm to get him to back off. That was where training paid off as we were able to calm them down, and after securing them to the rescue device tow them to shore. As we made headway toward the beach, the sweep funneled us back into the rip current, drawing us out again. This happened numerous times! The victims managed to hold on for "dear life" even though they swallowed a lot of salt water, were demoralized, and pummeled by the surf.

As time passed with each unsuccessful attempt to reach the shoreline, more people gathered to witness the rescue. At one point, there were about two hundred people glued to this emergency. Some of the patrons who knew the guards and witnessed this prolonged rescue became concerned. Finally, after many minutes of struggling to get the boys to shore, a lull in the waves gave us a chance to tow the boys to safety. We took advantage of this and hauled them to shore as fast as we could.

Although most rescues go unrecognized by beach patrons, this occasion was different. When we finally reached dry sand, they gave us a standing ovation. They were thrilled and relieved that everyone was safe after many minutes of horror. We were honored!

Once safely ashore, the boys collapsed on the wet sand. They were completely disorientated by their ordeal and it took them quite a while to catch their breath and regain their senses. Once recovered, they walked over, and thanked us for saving their lives. They were very appreciative and humbled by the sacrifice and risk made on their behalf. The boys then gathered their belongings and left the beach with, no doubt, a newfound respect for the Atlantic Ocean. It was, to say the least an experience I will remember for the rest of my life.

Chapter Four

The Emergence of Lifeguard Crews

As the turn-of-the-century approached, lifeguarding — and the valuable benefits it provided — was recognized up and down the coast. Most major resorts and even some of the smaller towns established lifeguards crews.

Because of their popularity and the benefits they provided, new rescue devices were experimented with and subsequently developed. That was the earmark for this era, development and refinement of lifesaving equipment as well as services. In Atlantic City and Cape May resorts, they extended service to the public by providing medical services, right along the beach. Hospital tents were the staple and were large canvas affairs that were hung over large wooden platforms. Inside a professional medical staff consisting of a doctor and nurse tended to the multitudes. Most problems, of course were routine and non-life threatening, such as a bad case of sunburn.

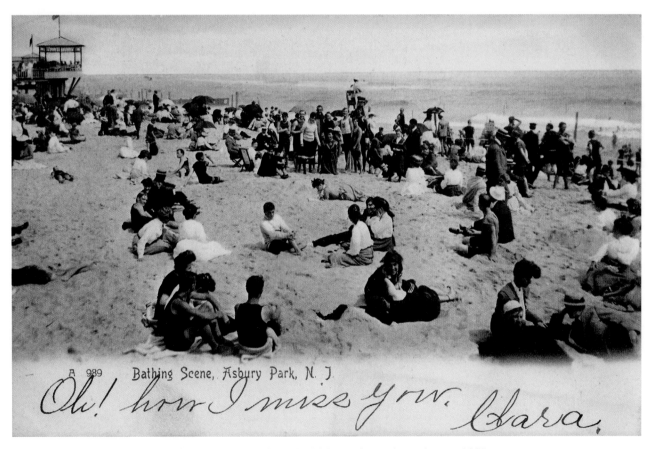

A typical 1900s beach scene at Asbury Park. The Asbury Park lifeguards are shown here in 1905.

There are lots of ways people can be injured at the beach. Splinters from the boardwalk were a popular malady of the day, as were scrapes and cuts from shells and rocks. More serious head and neck injuries could come from bathers or wave riders striking one of the poles used to support the bathing lines or — in what is still a problem to this day — people diving into the surf *head first* in water too shallow.

According to Margaret Thomas Bucholz, author of several New Jersey shore books, the first female lifeguard in New Jersey was hired in Surf City during World War II. According to a quote in the 1950s *Beachcomber*, a Long Beach Island newspaper: "Not all towns were able to guard their beaches. Surf City advertised for lifeguards for three sites on the ocean and one on the bay. A Beach Haven Terrace vacationer complained that the water was so warm it was a shame no lifeguard could be found. Surf City eventually settled for a girl: 'Have you noticed the very charming lifeguard at the bay bathing beach? Mary Wood is her name and she has won swimming medals in high school in Philadelphia. This can be a very difficult job for a girl and she needs the support of everyone that uses the bathing beach.'"

Early lifeguard crews were paid extraordinarily small sums to patrol the beach. In 1916, in Beach Haven, Alexander Ott, the first paid municipal employee, received a grand sum of $1.00 for the entire season to patrol the bathers! Apparently he was not stationed at the beach, but instead was expected to respond to emergencies.

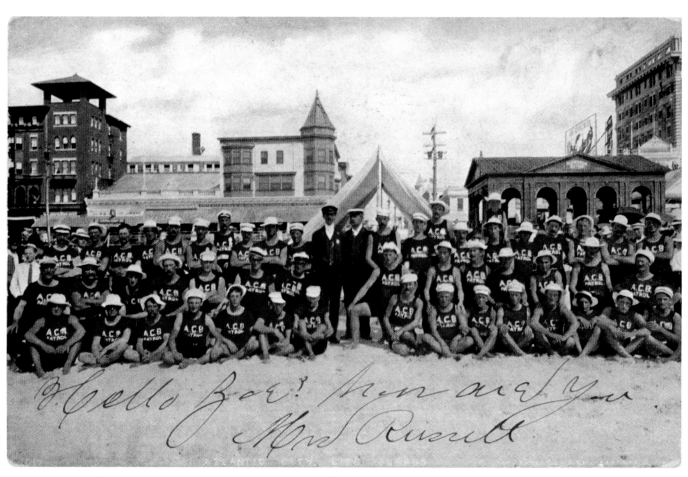

This is a rare 1902 colorized photo of the Atlantic City lifeguards. Note the "Constables of the Surf" aptly uniformed in the center.

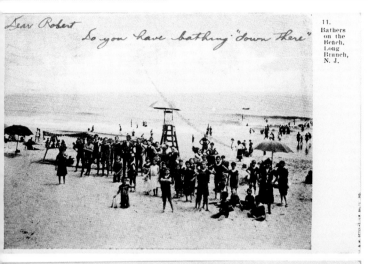

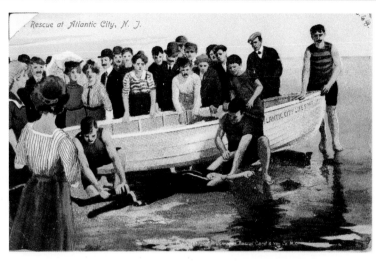

Developments were being made in the area of artificial respiration. Handed down from the Life-Saving Service, it was known in those days as "Resuscitation of the Apparently Drowned." The method was a far cry from the type of first aid administered by today's lifeguards.

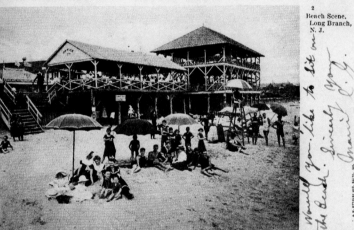

Lifeguards were referred to as "Beach Guards" in the older black and white version of the postcard. Here, Long Branch Lifeguards are shown in 1905 and 1907, respectively.

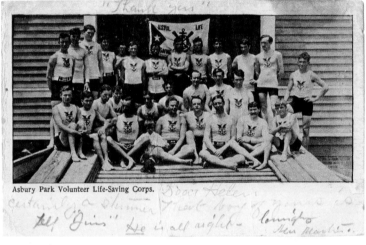

The volunteer lifesavers were founded around 1900 and, while it appeared that they assisted the lifeguards, it is thought that they were an adjunct to the Life-Saving Service that had a station at the east end of Deal Lake. This photo dates from 1905; the volunteers merged with the American Red Cross in 1913.
Courtesy of Asbury Park Library; Robert Stewart, Director.

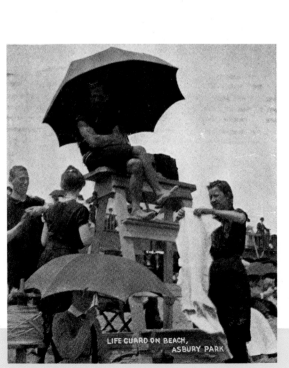

Asbury Park Lifeguards in 1906: note the age-old attraction of the male lifeguard to the female below. Lifeguard stands today often have perimeter ropes to prohibit patrons from distracting the guards.

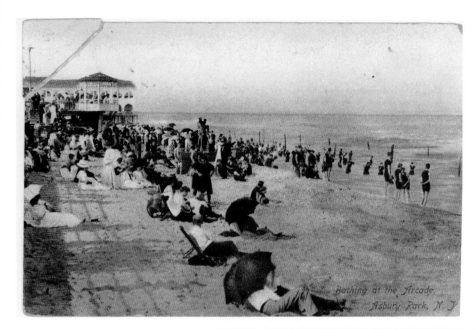

Bathing at the Arcade in
Asbury Park in 1909.

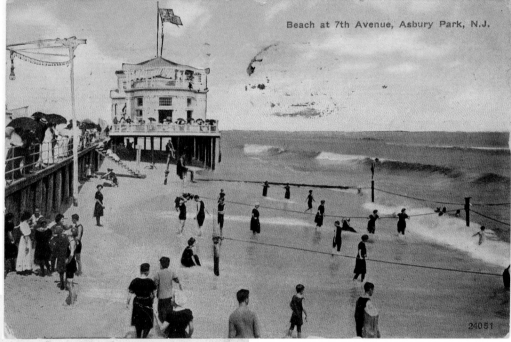

This rare, 1910 photo clearly
shows Asbury Park lifeguards
at Seventh Avenue observ-
ing bathers from chairs atop
poles. This practice was short
lived, perhaps only for several seasons. No photos after
1915 show this arrangement.

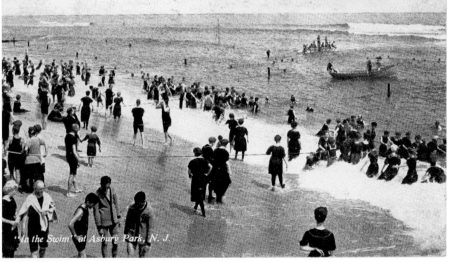

This 1909 photo shows Asbury Park
lifeguards patrolling from their boats
from inside the breakers and with patron
passengers. This practice would not be
considered wise by today's standards.

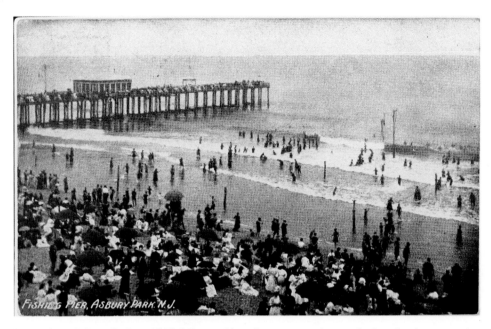

Low tide at Asbury Park in 1910. Lifeguard benches were in place at the beach adjacent to the fishing pier.

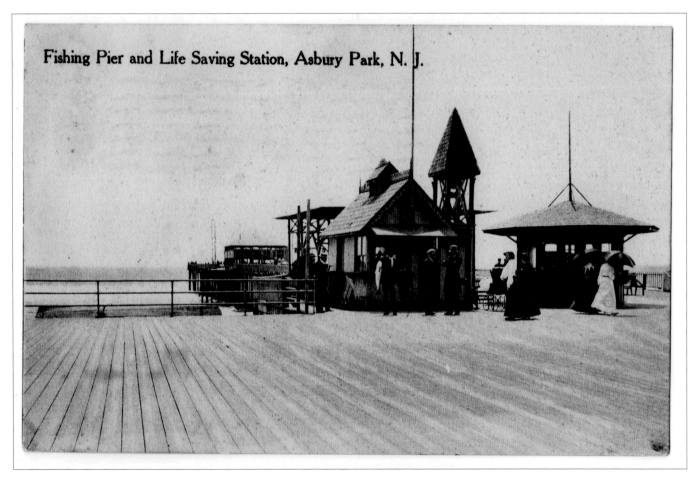

Fishing Pier and Life Saving Station, Asbury Park, N. J.

This rare, 1911 photo shows the Asbury Park Life Saving Station on the Boardwalk. Based on its location, it is surely the headquarters for the lifeguards. The inscription on the back reads: "The Life Savers are kept busy going out after people who go beyond their depth — with love, Aunt Clara." The often used and antiquated term "beyond their depth" today means people who are swept offshore in rip currents.

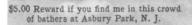

Bathers in Asbury Park in 1915. Note the lifeguard stand which is a platform mounted on a pole and shaded by a colorful umbrella. Note how many people are walking about the beach rather than lounging on chairs or towels as is common today.

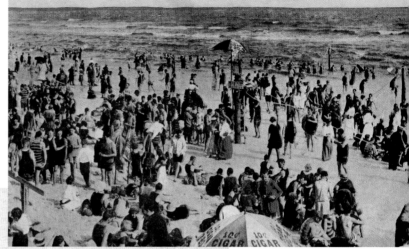

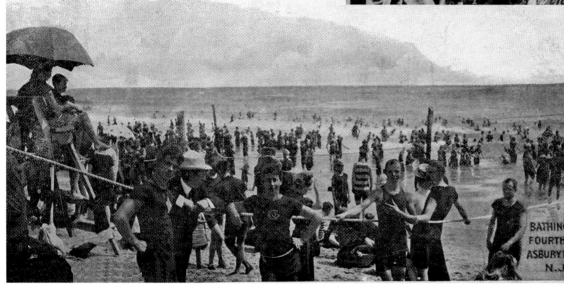

Lifeguards overseeing bathers at the Fourth Avenue beach in Asbury Park in 1913.

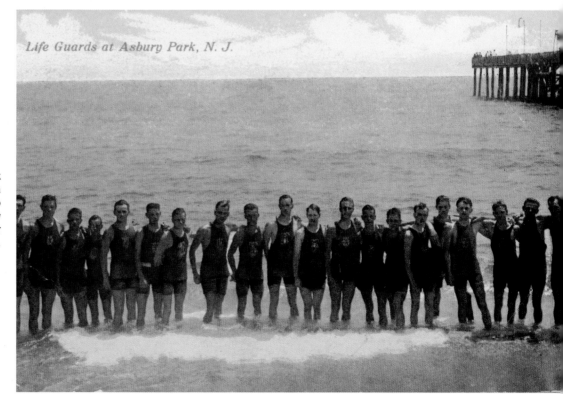

By 1913, the Asbury Park lifeguard crew had grown significantly in response to the increasing popularity of the city as a premier resort in New Jersey.

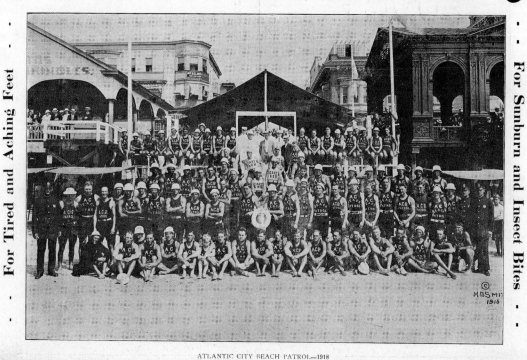

MENTHOLATUM

For Tired and Aching Feet

For Sunburn and Insect Bites

ATLANTIC CITY BEACH PATROL—1918

USED AND RECOMMENDED BY ALL LIFE GUARDS

The proud tradition of efficiency has become the landmark of the Atlantic City Beach Patrol. According to the ACLG Beneficial Association, "Not a man is permitted to don the red shirt until he has proved his metal (sic) in the rough seas with a boat and can buoy." This view of the Atlantic City Beach Patrol is in 1918 in an interesting sponsored postcard. The bold claim states it is used by "all" lifeguards.
From the Alfred M. Heston Collection,
Atlantic City Free Public Library.

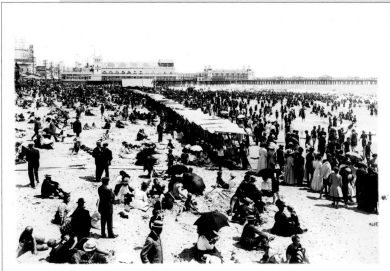

This crowded beach scene is from an undated postcard of Atlantic City. There is no doubt by the size of the crowd how popular a resort this city is and was.
Alfred M. Heston Collection,
Atlantic City Free Public Library.

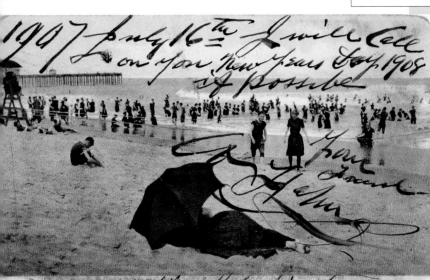

City of Long Branch Lifeguards are pictured here in 1907.

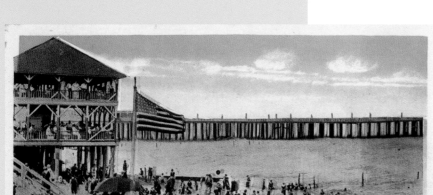

SCENE ON BEACH, LONG BRANCH, N. J.

Crowds continued to grow in Long Branch as pictured here in 1919 on a beach just south of the pier where steamships brought thousands to the Jersey Shore.

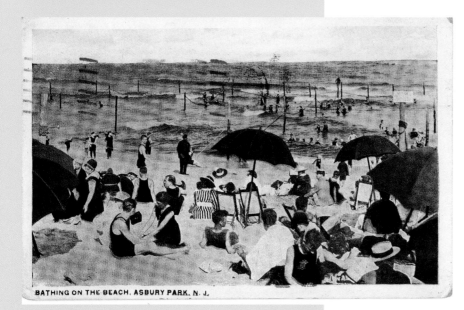

BATHING ON THE BEACH, ASBURY PARK, N. J.

Asbury Park bathers in 1919. Note the lifeguard "pole sitting." Bathing suits were rapidly becoming colorful and stylish, but there are quite a number of fully clothed patrons.

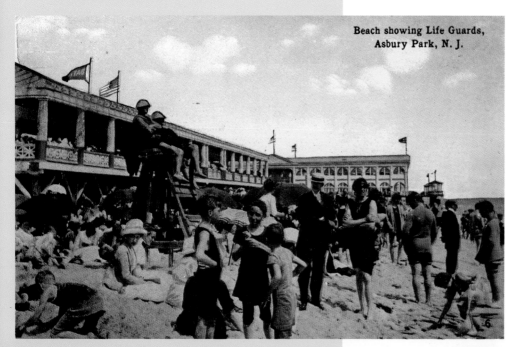

Beach showing Life Guards, Asbury Park, N. J.

This picture shows the popularity of Asbury Park as it rapidly grew into a shore resort. Their beaches were packed with tourists daily. Bathing suit styles would place this in the 1920s.

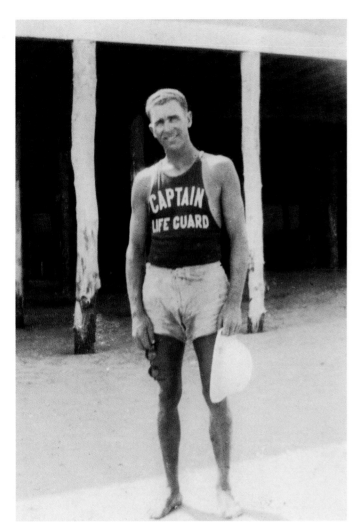

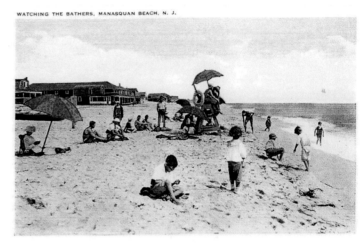

Rutherford Baker was Captain of the Cape May Beach Patrol in 1918. He was uncle to Jack Schellenger who later became Captain of the Cape May Beach Patrol. *Courtesy of Jack Schellenger.*

Manasquan Lifeguards were organized in the early 1930s and this is an early view circa 1930. *Courtesy of Mary Ware.*

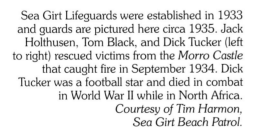

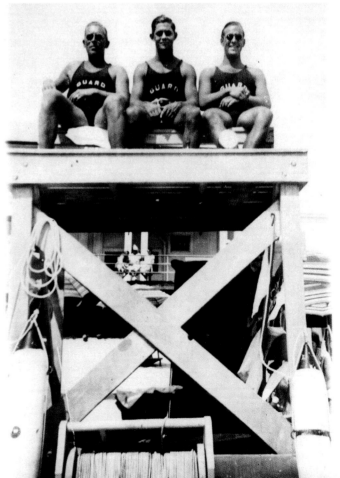

Sea Girt Lifeguards were established in 1933 and guards are pictured here circa 1935. Jack Holthusen, Tom Black, and Dick Tucker (left to right) rescued victims from the *Morro Castle* that caught fire in September 1934. Dick Tucker was a football star and died in combat in World War II while in North Africa. *Courtesy of Tim Harmon, Sea Girt Beach Patrol.*

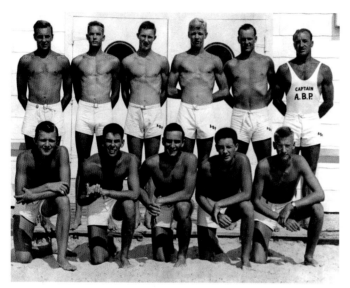

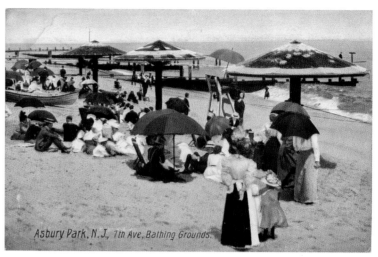

Colorful umbrellas shade visitors to Asbury Park in this undated photo, probably from the 1920s. Note the beach referred to as "bathing grounds."

Avalon Beach Patrol, established in 1905 is pictured here in 1939. Their present crew consists of ninety-five lifeguards patrolling 4.33 miles of beach from twenty-seven benches. *Courtesy of John Angemi, Jr.*

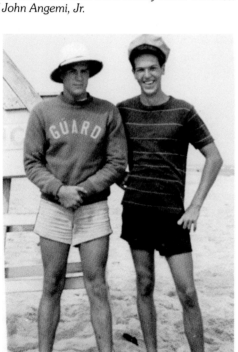

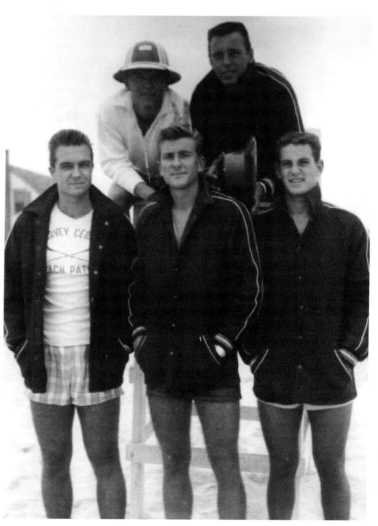

George Brewer, left, was Harvey Cedars' one lifeguard in 1942. When he had to report to the draft board, George Anger took his place on the 77th Street stand. Brother Jack, right, was Surf City's guard. During the World War II summers, the Harvey Cedars beach had a single guard—if one could be found. *Photo by Glenna Vreeland Wilcox; courtesy of Seasons in the Sun: A Photographic History of Harvey Cedars.*

Harvey Cedars Lifeguards in 1955. Top left to right: Bill Jaye, Michael Thomas; Bottom left to right: unknown, Ted Cedro, Pete Lyon. *Courtesy of Margaret Thomas Buchholz.*

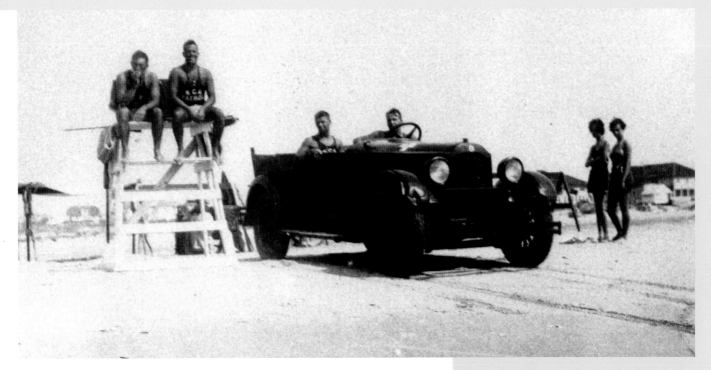

Wildwood guards in 1934 are pictured with their beach transportation. Note the admiring females to the right. *Courtesy of the Wildwood Historical Society.*

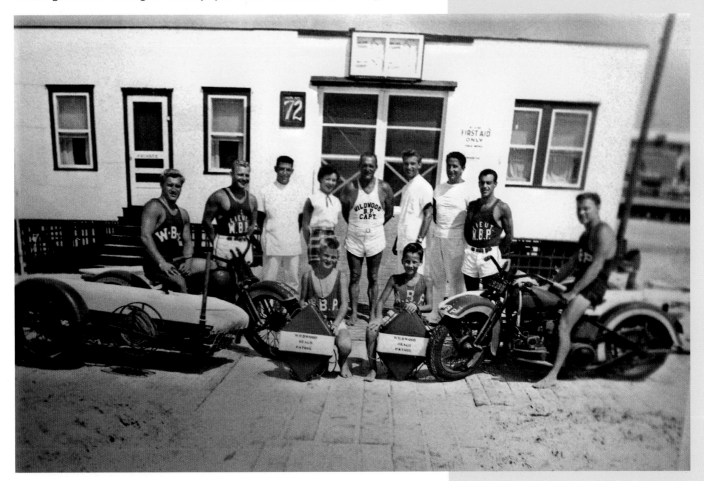

Wildwood Beach Patrol used motorcycles with sidecars to cover their wide beaches. Several guards with their bikes are shown outside Patrol Headquarters. Note the junior lifeguards with the diamond cans. *Courtesy of the Wildwood Historical Society.*

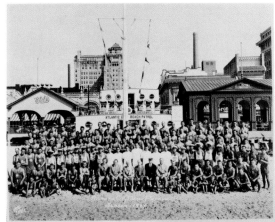

Team photo of the Atlantic City Beach Patrol in 1949. The crew had grown substantially in number based on the popularity of the resort.
From the Alfred M. Heston Collection, Atlantic City Free Public Library.

This practice was known as "pole sitting," a job usually reserved for rookie lifeguards. Some patrols called for guards to sit on the outermost southern pole during peak hours as the prevailing wind blew in from the southeast. Patrons would playfully jump on the bathing ropes in an attempt to shake the pole and dislodge the guard.

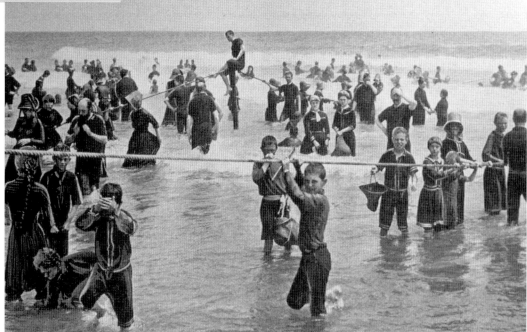

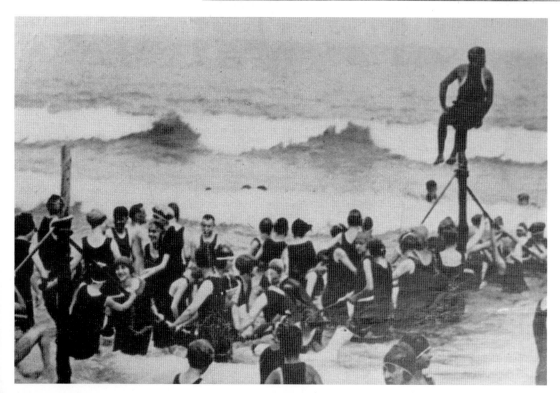

Rare photo of a lifeguard pole sitting in Asbury Park in 1924.

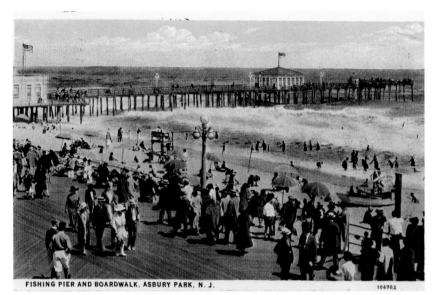

FISHING PIER AND BOARDWALK, ASBURY PARK, N. J.

Asbury Park Lifeguards by the fishing pier in 1927. Note the surfboat at the ready.

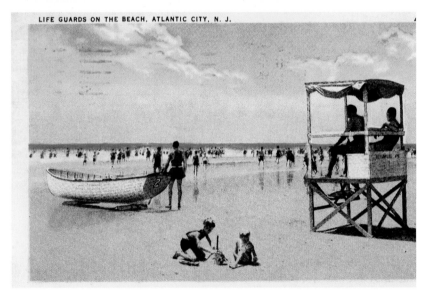

LIFE GUARDS ON THE BEACH, ATLANTIC CITY, N. J.

Atlantic City Lifeguards in 1935 maintain a vigilant watch over their patrons.

Asbury Park Lifeguards in 1936. Their uniforms had become a daring red and their benches were now platforms, painted green and similar to the design used in Spring Lake today.

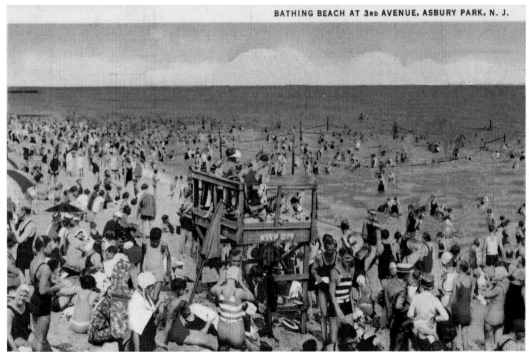

BATHING BEACH AT 3RD AVENUE, ASBURY PARK, N. J.

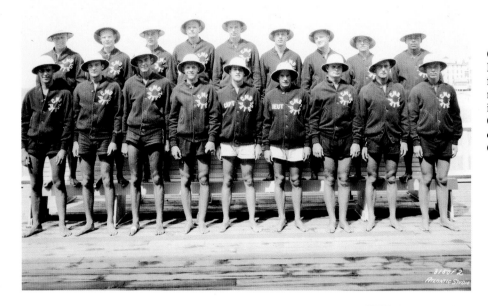

Cape May Beach Patrol circa 1935. Front row, Jack Schellenger is third from the right. Notice the pith helmets, which were similar to those issued to the United States Navy Construction Battalions (Seabees) during World War II.
Courtesy of Jack Schellenger.

Cape May Beach Patrol lifeguards Walton, Homan, and Hunt (first names unknown) are pictured with their equipment in 1940.
Courtesy of Buzz Mogck.

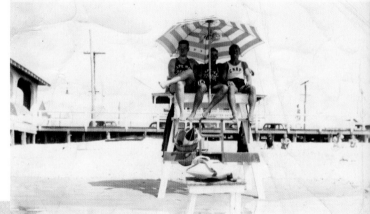

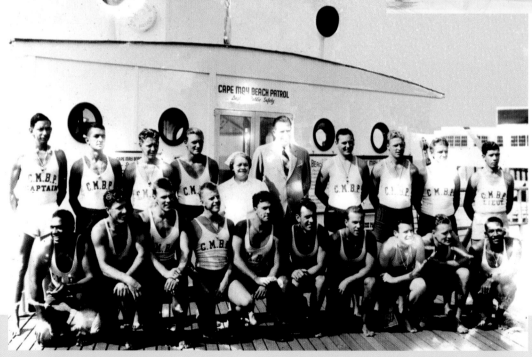

Cape May lifeguards were first hired in 1911 with Tom Keenan serving as the first captain of the Beach Patrol. Early rules for the well disciplined crew included "shirts worn at all times" and "no talking to girls for more than a few minutes." The team photo is of Cape May Beach Patrol circa 1950.
Courtesy of Buzz Mogck.

Cape May Beach Patrol poses proudly in their classic red tank tops. Registered nurse Ida Stevens became a twenty plus-year veteran of the patrol until the city eliminated her position. *Courtesy of Buzz Mogck.*

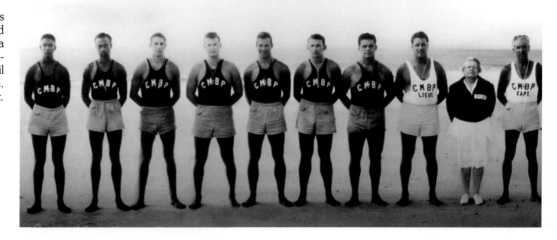

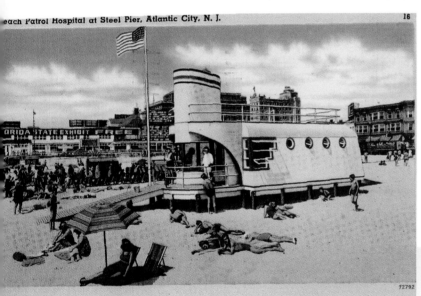

The art deco design of the Atlantic City Beach Patrol's headquarters is certainly novel by today's standards. Similar design applications can be seen in the lifeguard stands in Miami's Southbeach section.

Avon-by-the-Sea Lifeguards in the 1930s. Their crew was established in 1929. Jim Kirk is second from left, Milt Hamilton is fifth from left, and lifeguard captain Tom Child is at the right end. The police badges pinned to their belts shows they were sworn in as police officers. *Courtesy of Kenneth Child.*

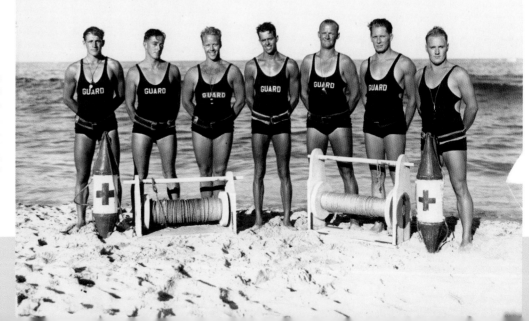

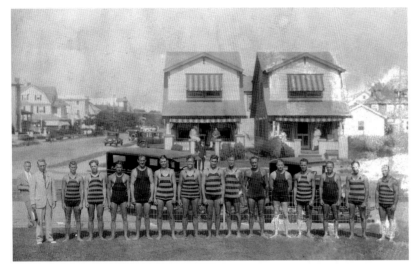

This rare and partly damaged photo shows the Bradley Beach Lifeguards in their unique striped tank tops sometime in the 1930s. Lettering indicates they were employed by the "Department of Public Safety." *Courtesy of Dick Johnson.*

The first paid crew in Long Beach Township Beach Patrol, currently the largest crew in New Jersey is pictured here in 1936. Their volunteer patrol started in 1933. *Courtesy of Long Beach Township Beach Patrol.*

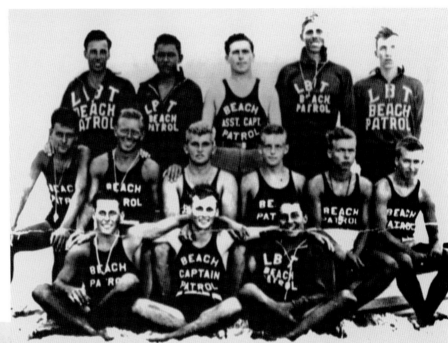

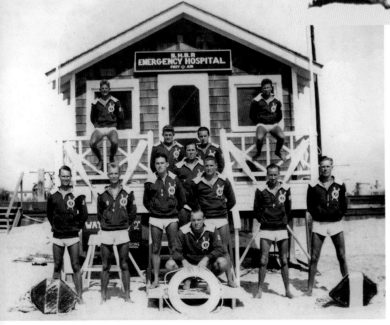

Stone Harbor Beach Patrol was established in 1912. They are pictured by their headquarters in 1939. They are equipped with diamond rescue cans and a ring buoy. *Courtesy of Captain Sandy Bosacco.*

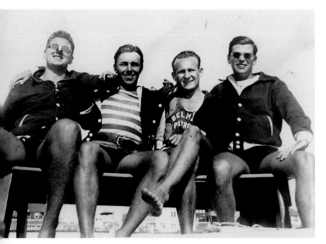

Belmar lifeguards pose on 4th Avenue in 1941.
Courtesy of Bob Watkins, Jr.

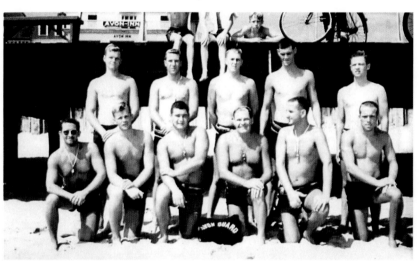

Avon Lifeguards, here with Howard Rowland (bottom row, third from right) are pictured again in 1956. Also shown are Dr. Joseph Jasaitis, top row left and his brother John, bottom row, second from left. Also pictured is Avon icon Dr. James Forsyth, bottom row left who was both a physician and attorney. Many Boy Scouts under his leadership became lifeguards. *Courtesy of Joseph Jasaitis.*

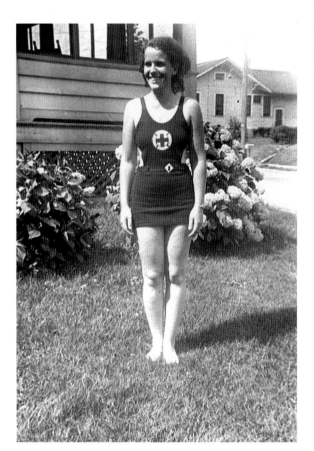

The first female lifeguard in Lavallette was Carol MacKinnon, pictured here in 1940. Note the Red Cross logo on her suit. She is the aunt of author Michael Fowler. *Courtesy of Gordon Hesse.*

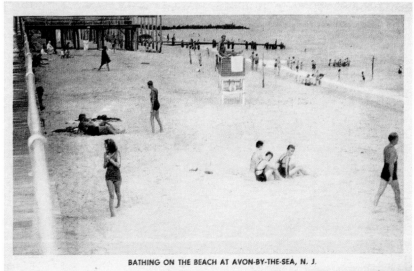

BATHING ON THE BEACH AT AVON-BY-THE-SEA, N. J.

Woodland Avenue Beach in Avon-by-the-Sea is shown in this 1938 view. The lifeguard stand is an elevated platform on which the guards would place beach chairs. Windbreakers could be wound around the upper part of the frame to shield the guards.

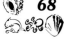

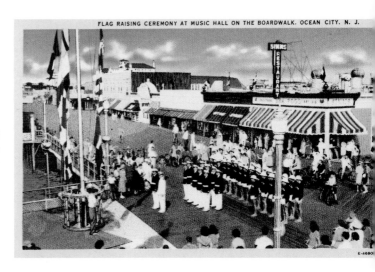

Ocean City Beach Patrol at its morning flag raising ceremony.

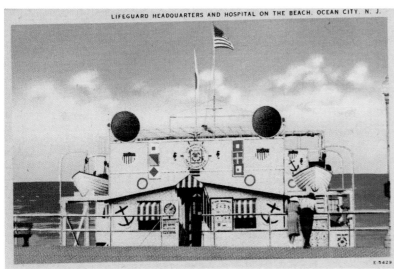

Ocean City Beach Patrol headquarters at 10th Street was constructed to look like the bridge of an ocean liner. It was constructed in the 1920s and wiped out in a storm in 1962.

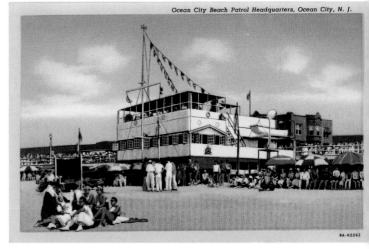

The 10th Street Ocean City Beach Patrol headquarters as constructed after the 1962 storm.

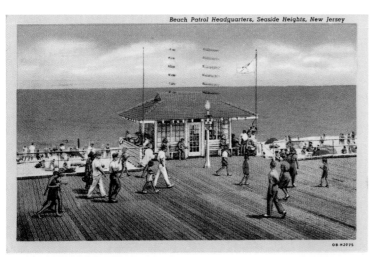

Seaside Heights Beach Patrol Headquarters circa 1948.

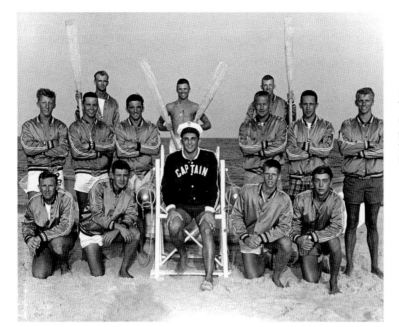

Lavallette Beach Patrol in 1952. They currently patrol 1.5 miles of beach from nine ocean lifeguard stands and two at the bay with their thirty-six lifeguards. *Courtesy of Gordon Hesse.*

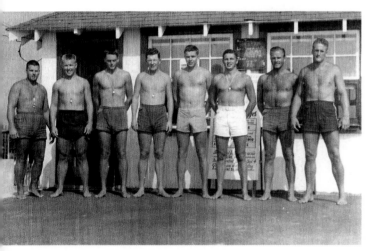

Manasquan Lifeguards proudly pose by their headquarters in 1950. *Courtesy of Mary Ware.*

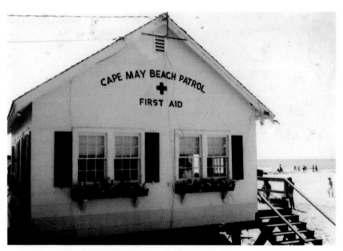

This is the third version of Cape May Beach Patrol's four headquarters. The first, located at Stockton Avenue, was constructed from the wheelhouse of a ship and is pictured earlier in the chapter. *Courtesy of Jack Schellenger.*

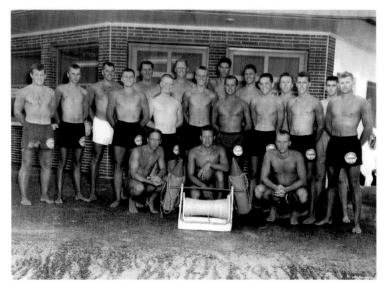

A photo taken at least a decade later reveals a much larger crew outside the new headquarters for the Manasquan Lifeguards. *Courtesy of Mary Ware.*

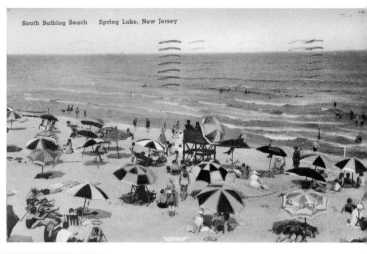

Spring Lake Lifeguards in 1940 with their platform style benches, which still exist to this day. In 1907, a bath house set out bathing poles between Newark and Brighton Avenues and a single lifeguard was hired after funds were raised. He was equipped with a surfboat.

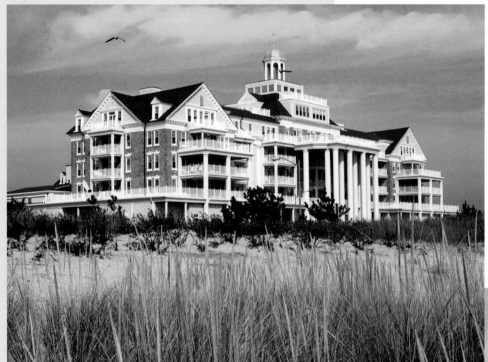

Early visitors to Spring Lake might have stayed in luxurious hotels such as the Essex and Sussex, constructed in 1914. At 2:15 p.m. on July 1, 1916, young Charles Bruder, an employee of the hotel, was fatally attacked by a shark. Veteran Spring Lake lifeguards Captain George White and Chris Anderson rowed to Bruder and pulled him into their surfboat. Both of his legs had been torn off just below the knee.

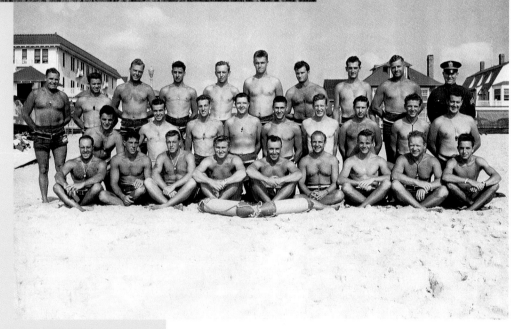

Belmar lifeguards in 1947 with lifeguard legend Howard Rowland, standing at left. All Belmar team photos were taken on 10th Avenue, a tradition existing today. *Courtesy of Bob Watkins.*

Modern Lifeguards

Lifeguards of the twenty-first century play a similar, yet more refined role than their predecessors. New requirements and certifications have made the job much more rigorous. Beach supervisors view the job as risk and liability management rather than a crew just watching over bathers. Litigation and lawsuits have made the job demanding — where less than a one hundred percent success rate is not acceptable. Paperwork and documentation is critical.

There are three basic philosophies of modern lifeguarding and what is adopted is largely a part of the beach's location. Each has its merits and flaws. In New Jersey, where swimming areas are confined, guards adopt a preventive philosophy. They will prevent bathers from entering dangerous waters and "herd" or move them about as conditions warrant. Where crowds are massive and crowd control is difficult, if not impossible, as on some of New York's beaches, guards are reactive — they will react to emergencies as they happen. In California, where beaches are expansive, some agencies adopt the patrol philosophy — they cover the beaches in 4WD vehicles and stand ready for radio calls to emergencies, much like police departments.

There is a difference between lifeguarding — preventing bathers from becoming victims — and lifesaving — rescuing victims in trouble. Lifeguards are trained observers who are responsible for overseeing the health and welfare of bathers. Their job is demanding. They must identify rip currents, spot potential victims, plan and execute rescues, engage in preventive actions, locate lost patrons, direct and manage large crowds, administer first aid, document training and emergency actions, maintain advanced certifications, participate in physical conditioning as well as rig and maintain all the equipment lifeguards use. Lifeguards are the insurance policy for the agency that hires them. Some supervisors don't view it as a job of "lifeguarding," but as risk and liability management.

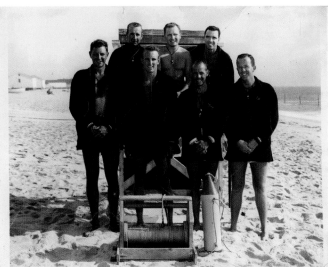

Risden's Beach Lifeguards pose by their rescue reel and rescue torpedo at Point Pleasant Beach in 1953. Veteran lifeguard Gene Leahy is seated at the top right.
Courtesy of Dr. Eugene Leahy.

A Bradley Beach lifeguard is surrounded by beach patrons as he stands at the bow of a Hankin's skiff. The picture appears to be from the 1950s or early 1960s.

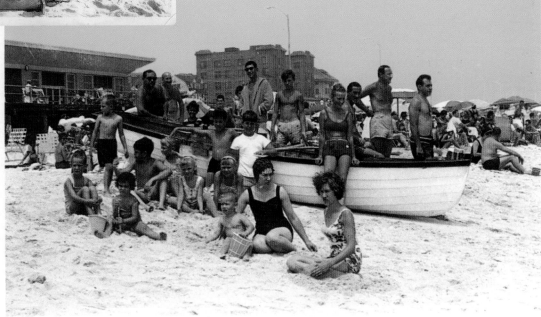

Having Fun at Bradley Beach, New Jersey

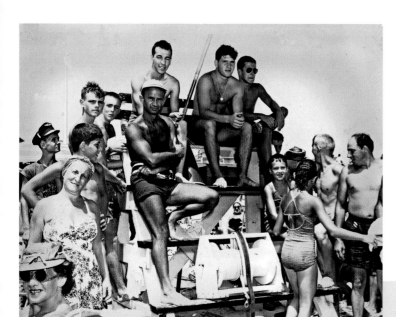

In 1953, the Bradley Beach Lifeguards staged a strike and were replaced by an "Emergency Squad" consisting of police officers and towns-people. The McCabe Avenue crew is shown surrounded by supportive beach patrons. *Courtesy of Dick Johnson.*

This 1962 team photo shows the Belmar life-guards with shore no-tables Howard Rowland (front row with pith hel-met), Ray Darby (front row, second from right), and eventual leader of the crew Joe Semas (back row, right end).

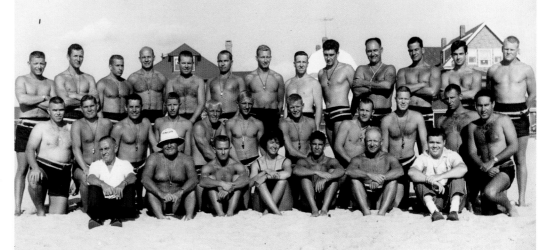

The smallest municipal lifeguard crew in New Jersey is in the Village of Loch Arbor where six lifeguards patrol a small bathing area along a three hundred-foot beach. This compares to Long Beach Township's crew of 213 guards along twelve miles of beach. This picture is from 1973. *Courtesy of John McCahill.*

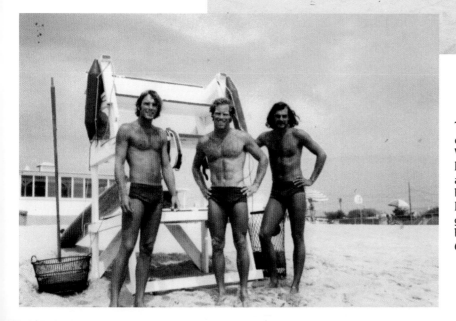

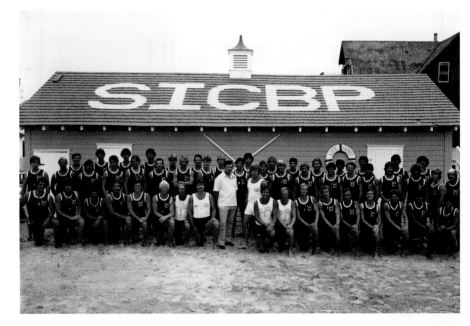

Sea Isle City Beach patrol in 1980. The photo was taken on 44th Street in Sea Isle. *Courtesy of Dr. Thomas P. McCann.*

Lifeguards are often faced with hazardous situations. There were fifteen drownings during the summer of 1995. *Courtesy of Asbury Park Press, a Gannet Co. newspaper.*

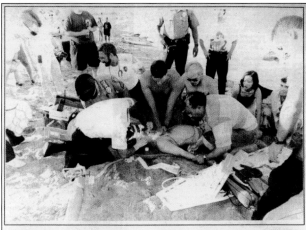

Tragedy at Beach

VACATIONER DROWNS. SEE PAGE 2 FOR STORY

Asbury Park Press Friday, Aug. 18, 1995

HURRICANE FELIX: Tragedy strikes Shore area

3 die in treacherous surf

From page **A1**

the boys as Jaleel, 13, and Hafiz Abdul-Majeed, 11. Their father, Akram Abdul-Majeed, brought the two boys and two younger siblings from their home in Irvington for a day at the beach.

A little girl, another child and the father, wrapped in a blanket over his drenched jeans, were escorted from the beach shortly after the first boy was found. The immediate family was notified of the drownings last night, and DiCorcia said a boardwalk homeowner had allowed the boys' relatives to stay in the house during the search.

The boys' father had been sitting near the ocean when the children were dragged into the water and he immediately ran in after them, DiCorcia said. The man was unable to reach the boys and was pulled from the

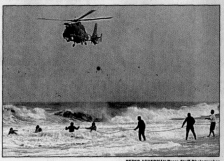

PETER ACKERMAN/Press Staff Photographer

● A Coast Guard helicopter and rescuers search for two boys who were swept into the ocean yesterday off Point Pleasant Beach.

The summer of 1995 was one of the most deadly for the Jersey Shore with a total of fifteen drownings over the summer. Fourteen of them occurred after hours or on unguarded beaches. *Courtesy of Asbury Park Press, a Gannet Co. newspaper.*

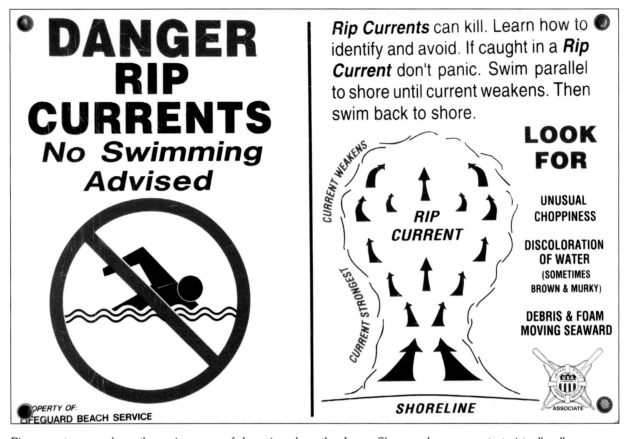

Rip currents are perhaps the major cause of drowning along the Jersey Shore and are present at virtually all beaches. Lifeguard agencies post signs to warn the bathing public, especially for those foolish enough to bathe on unprotected beaches or before or after guarded hours.

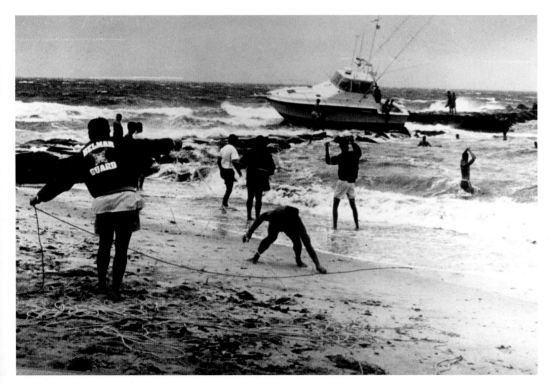

Belmar Lifeguards rescued everyone aboard this floundering boat that came up on the jetty during a nor'easter. *Courtesy of Beverly Streeter.*

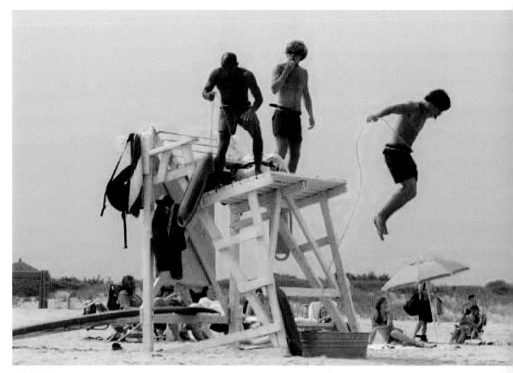

Sandy Hook Lifeguards at Gateway National Recreation Area initiate a rescue. *Courtesy of Dave Pearson.*

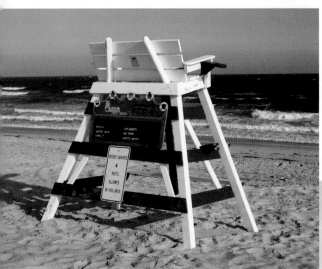

Colorful lifeguard stands dot the Jersey Shore. This one is in Cape May.

Women have played an increasingly important role in ocean lifeguarding. It started in the 1940s with a shortage of men due to the war effort. Many were hired in the 1960s and have been increasing in numbers ever since. Sandy Hook's 2007 crew is pictured here. *Courtesy of Dave Pearson.*

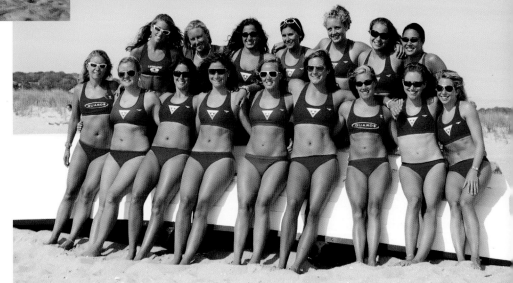

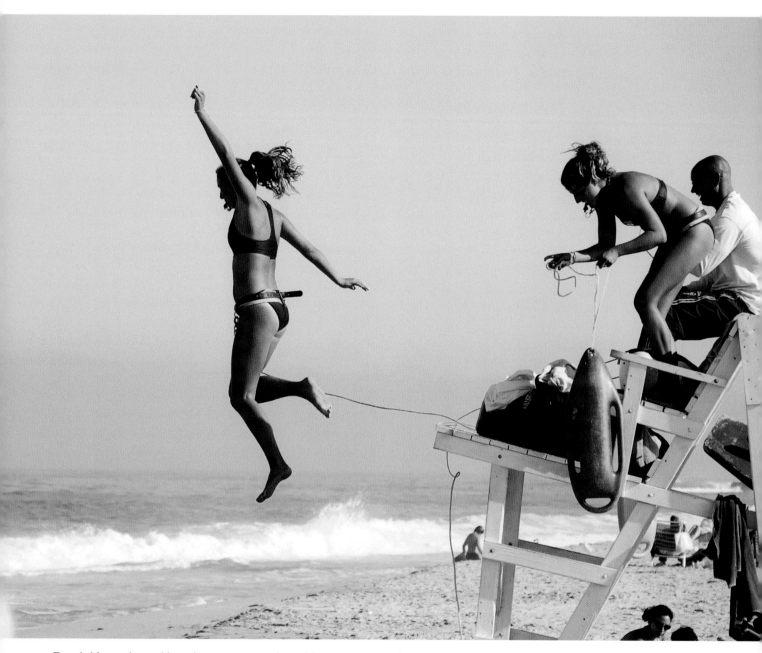

Female lifeguards are able and competent members of the rescue crew and an entire tournament is dedicated to their athletic prowess each year at the All Women's tournament at Sandy Hook. *Photo Courtesy of Dave Pearson.*

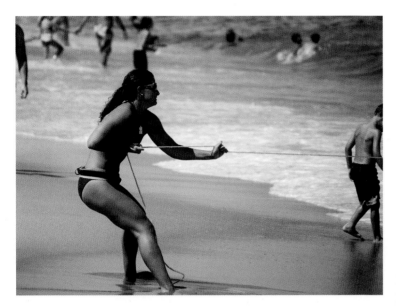

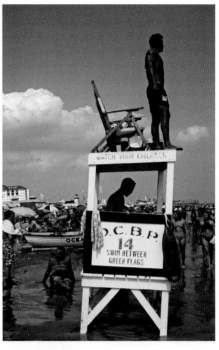

Female lifeguard making a line rescue at Sandy Hook. Notice how beachgoers seem oblivious to the saving of a person's life. Guards consider this all in a day's work. *Courtesy of Dave Pearson.*

Ocean City uses a two-tier stand to tend to their bathers.

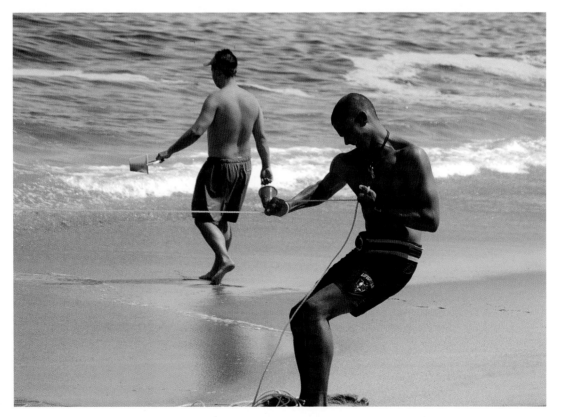

Sandy Hook Lifeguards in action during a line rescue. *Courtesy of Dave Pearson.*

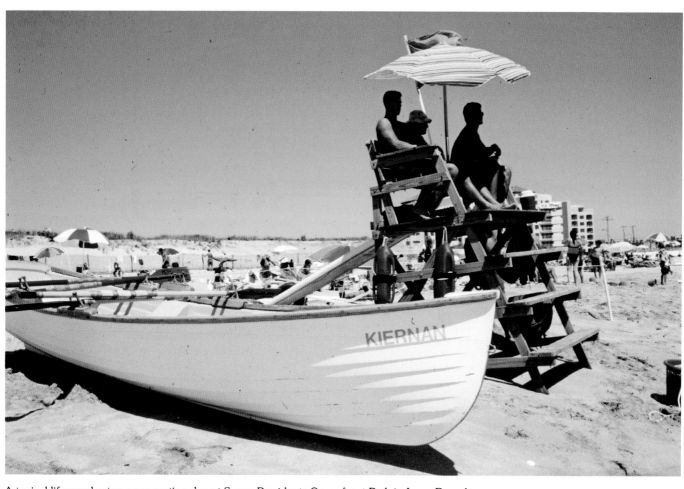

A typical lifeguard setup on a routine day at Seven Presidents Oceanfront Park in Long Branch.
A Van Duyne skiff can be seen in the foreground.

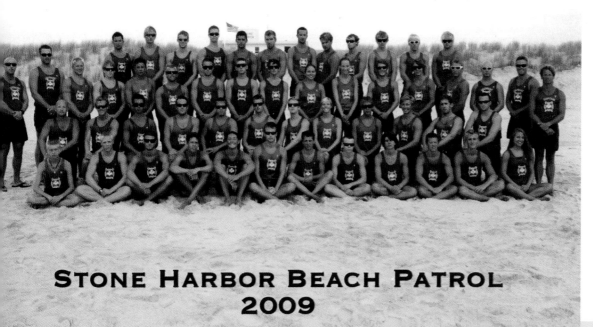

The Stone Harbor Beach Patrol was established in 1912 and presently employs about sixty lifeguards. They patrol 2.3 miles of beach from twenty-one lifeguard stands.

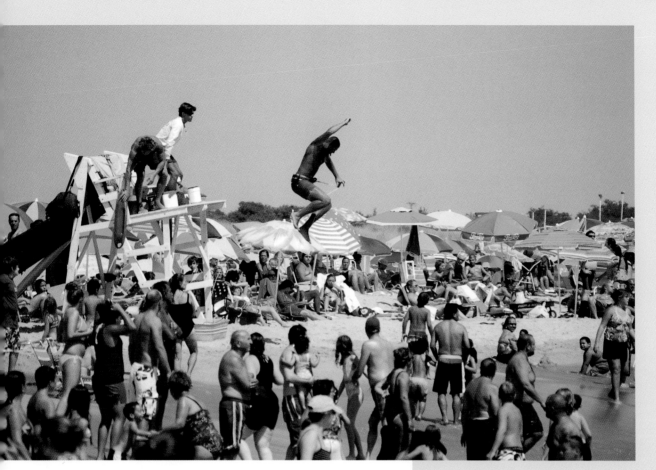

Sandy Hook lifeguards blast into action during a line rescue. *Courtesy of Dave Pearson.*

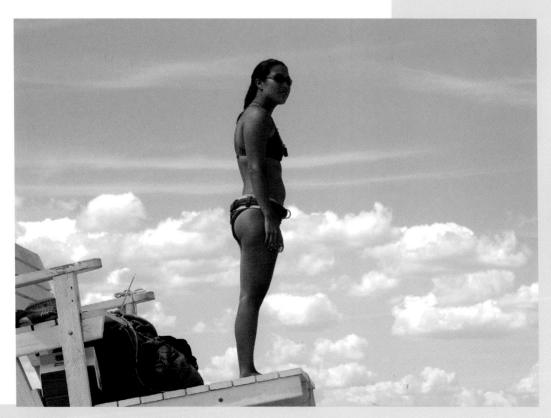

At the most fundamental level, lifeguards are paid observers of bathers. Victim identification is perhaps the most challenging aspect of ocean lifeguarding and certainly one of the most difficult concepts to teach new recruits. *Courtesy of Dave Pearson.*

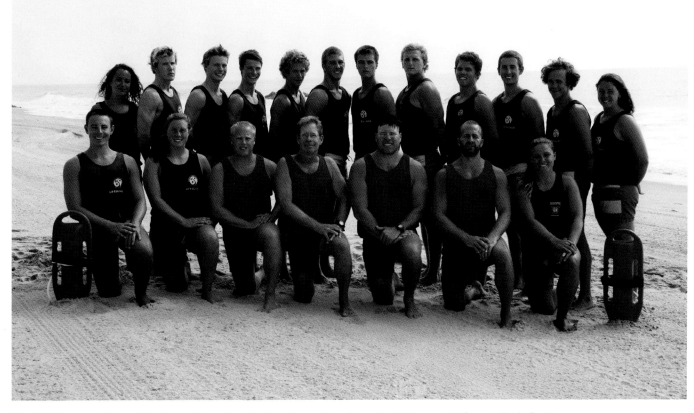

The 2009 crew at Seven Presidents Oceanfront Park in Long Branch, part of Monmouth County Park System. Authors Ted Olsen and Spike Fowler are in the front row (to the left in red).

My First Rescue

Michael "Spike" Fowler,
Lifeguard Supervisor
Monmouth County Park System

My first rescue was an embarrassment. It was during the summer of 1964 in Avon-by-the-Sea where I had been hired as a rookie. I was only on the job for a week or so and I hadn't received much training at all, especially in "victim identification," now considered one of the most important components.

I was assigned to the Woodland Avenue Beach with my more experienced partner, Richie Crocker. Despite very bad water conditions, he decided to get breakfast at Skopas, the nearby pavilion. He told me he'd be right there for me if I needed him and then left me alone on the stand. The water was rough, with rip currents everywhere. People were bathing in what I perceived to be normal, but rough conditions. There were two or three people swimming when suddenly a beach patron came running up to me and said, "Those people are

in trouble!" They looked OK to me, but I grabbed the rescue can, clipped it to my belt (we used the canvas and leather rescue belts at the time) and ran into the water to help them, along with the beach patron. Luckily, everyone was brought to shore safely just in time to see Richie Crocker running down the beach with food all over his face. The patron and I had made the rescue!

The rescue was over, but the patron screamed and ranted at me: "You shouldn't be a lifeguard — don't you know what you're doing?" Other beach patrons were there to witness my scolding. I was shattered and considered quitting right on the spot from my shame.

I didn't though. I stuck it out, eventually going on to make hundreds of successful rescues and supervising and witnessing thousands more. What I didn't realize at the time is that people in trouble are always swimming, at least at first! The difference is, they're swimming west, but heading east — off shore.

I'll never forget that day and how upset I was with Crocker for hanging me out like that. From that point forward, I always knew when someone was in trouble.

Chapter Five

Lifeguard Rescue Gear

Lifeguards, like all other public safety agencies, have tools of the trade that have developed over the decades.

Lifeguard Boats

Patrol and rescue surfboats were the staple of lifeguards from the beginnings of beach patrols. The seaworthy skiffs were rowed offshore beyond the breakers to keep a watchful eye over bathers. If someone were swept offshore, they were hoisted into the boat and taken to shore. These boats played a key role in the development of lifeguarding. Boat crews were admired for their bravado and surf skill. It takes a certain kind of lifeguard willing to row a boat out through heavy breakers.

In general, boats are classic Jersey skiffs, approximately sixteen feet in length with a four-foot or slightly wider beam. They are lapstrake design with the boards overlapping up to the gunwale. There, two sets of oar or rowlocks are anchored to the top rail. The oars are usually 8' to 8 1/2' in length and the boat has two seats for the rowers, usually a rear or stern seat and some even have a small bow seat. The classic boats were constructed from Jersey cedar and/or plywood and in later years with fiberglass.

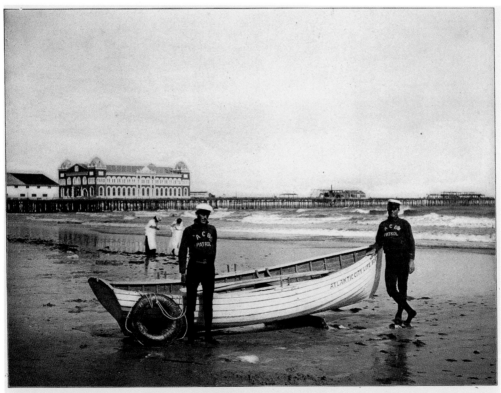

LIFE GUARD ON THE BEACH

Atlantic City Lifeguards by their rescue boat in this early 1900s photo. Modesty standards of the day required full woolen suits which were slow to dry and uncomfortable. The design of the skiff is exactly the same as modern lifeguard boats.

There are several boat builders of note. Charles E. Hankins of Lavallette built many lifeguard skiffs primarily for beaches in Ocean and Monmouth County. Charles Morgan Hankins established the Boatworks, located along Grand Central Avenue, in 1912 and the business was passed down to his sons, Charles and James. Sturdy and seaworthy are the reputation of the Hankins' skiff. Some of their boats became high-speed rumrunners during Prohibition although they were also known for their pound boats and pleasure boats.

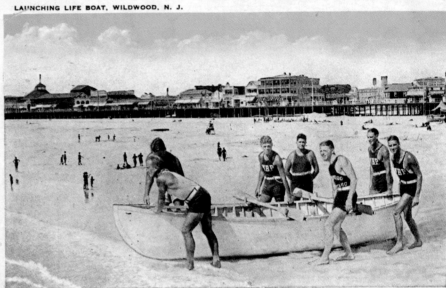

Lifeguards prepare to launch a surfboat in Wildwood.

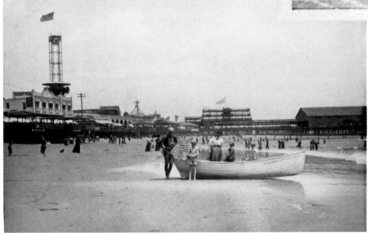

A family poses in the surfboat in Atlantic City, taken most likely in the 1920s. The 16-foot wooden Jersey skiff is a classic design.

Surfboats played a significant role in rescues, particularly in the early days of lifeguarding.

SAVED SIX FROM DROWNING

An Entire Family Saved From a Watery Grave at Cape May Yesterday.

Six persons were rescued from drowning at Cape May yesterday. Rev. W. V. Liebhart, pastor of the Moravian church at Bethlehem, Pa., and his three daughters, Anna, Ethel and Helen, were in bathing. The last named was being taught to swim by F. C. Hall, of Washington.

The young woman thought she could swim alone and tried to do so. Then she became frightened and called for help. Her father, who was near by, and the two other sisters, also Mr. Hall, went to the rescue.

All got beyond their depth. The lifeguard boat moved quickly toward them, saving the five by pulling them in and bringing them ashore. All were in an unconscious condition and required medical attention.

The sixth person saved was a man who held to an iron pier support until the lifeboat came.

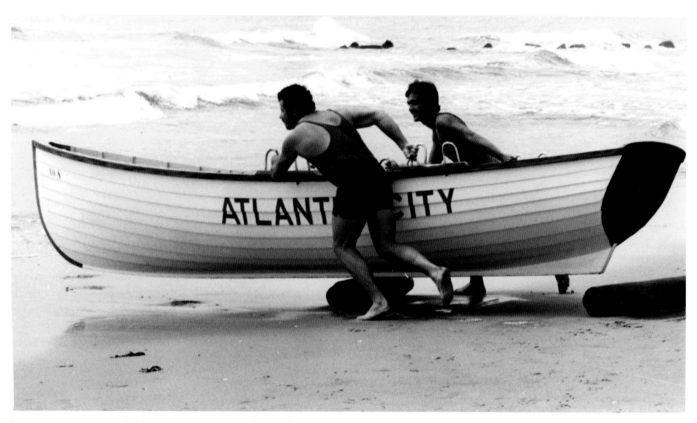

Most certainly taken in the 1960s, two members of the Atlantic City Beach Patrol launch a Van Sant wooden skiff. Note the rounded rowlocks that hold the oars in place. Many injuries occurred on older style rowlocks that had pointed ends. *Alfred M. Heston Collection – Atlantic City Free Public Library.*

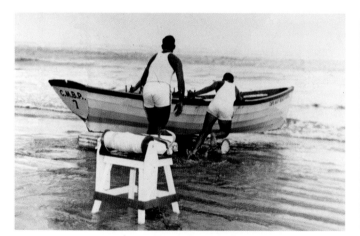

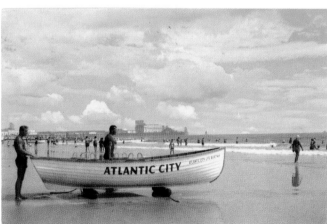

Cape May lifeguards launching their surfboat off boat rollers.
A rescue reel with line is in the foreground.

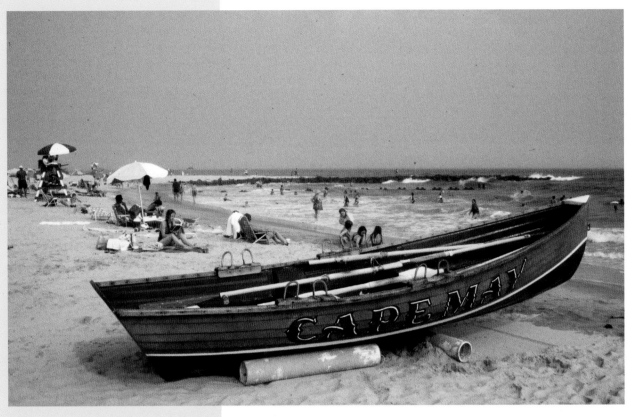

Colorful markings on a Van Duyne fiberglass surfboat at Cape May make them distinctive from other beach patrol's boats.

Cape May lifeguards are shown with a locally constructed skiff made by Pharo Boat Works and Marina. Rollers constructed with firing strips helped with moving the boat through the sand. Note the front decking and thole pins as rowlocks on this surfboat.

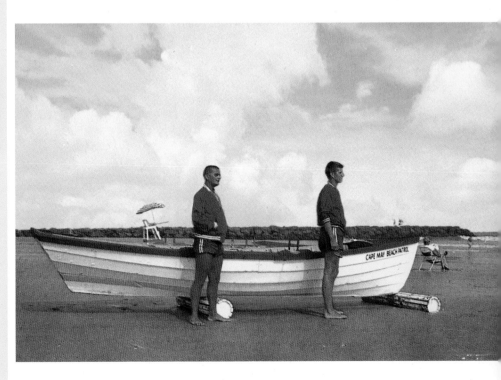

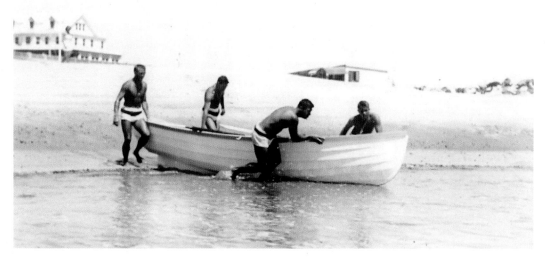

Allenhurst lifeguards, including Harry Hoehn launch a Hankins surfboat. *Courtesy of Harry Hoehn.*

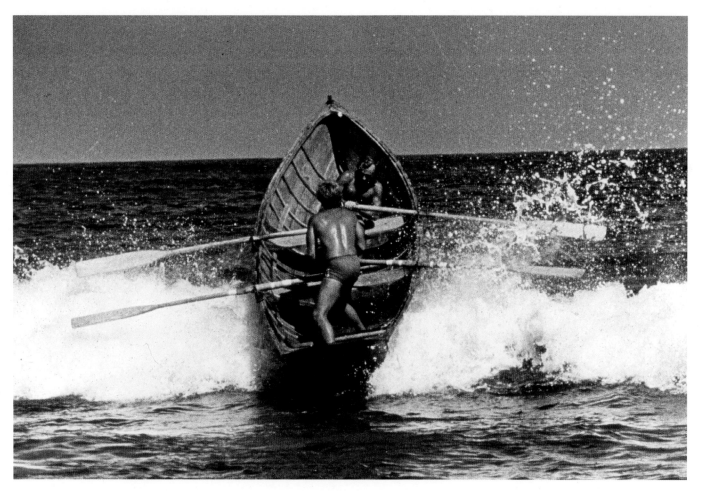

Monmouth County Lifeguards are the only crews in the United States to still employ the standup rowing style. This sixteen-foot Hankin's skiff is quite seaworthy. Author Michael Fowler is standing at the stern position with lifeguard Howard Hardie at the bow oars. The photo likeness became a logotype for many lifeguard designs on tournament t-shirts. *Courtesy of Robert Longo.*

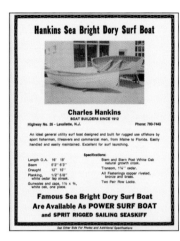

Renowned boat builder Charles Hankins from Lavallette used these flyers to promote his line of surfboats which became the standard along the Jersey Shore. They were extremely sturdy and seaworthy.

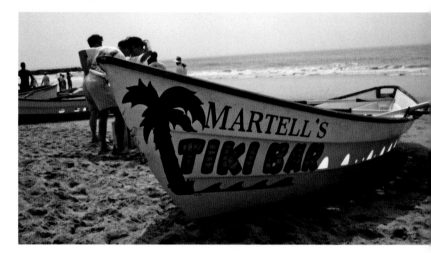

Newer models of surfboats are constructed of fiberglass and are self bailing. Any water coming into the boat will quickly empty through the holes in the hull. The floor decking is slightly above the waterline.

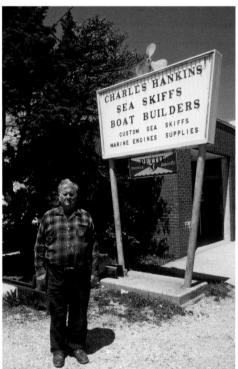

Charles Hankins outside his Lavallette boatworks. His name is synonymous with quality lifeguard skiffs.

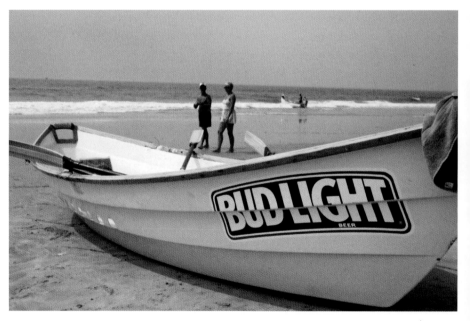

The Schock Dories, constructed in California compete against the Asay boats in the competitive boat market. Some of them, such as the one pictured here have national sponsors.

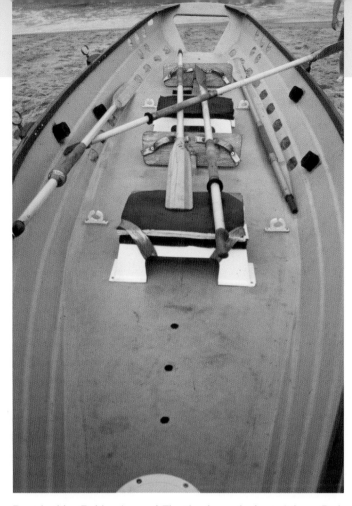

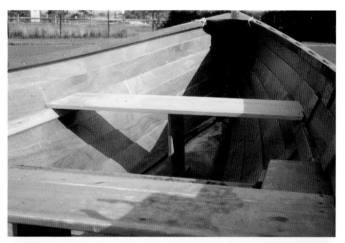

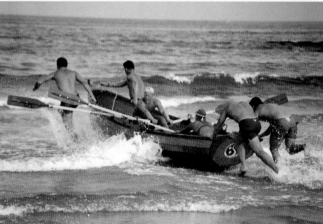

Boat builder Bobby Asay of Florida, formerly from Asbury Park constructs the fastest competitive surfboats in the United States. Note the selfbailing and fiberglass construction.

Bob Asay successfully experimented with a rib-less design, previously unheard of in the construction of lapstrake boats. This made the boat significantly lighter and faster.

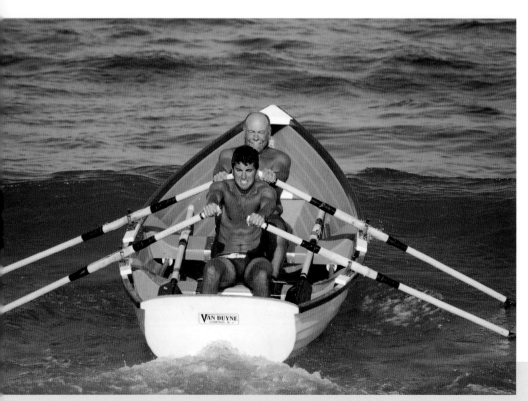

The most popular boat along the Jersey Coast is the Van Duyne. Molded in fiberglass in classic Jersey skiff design, the boat is seaworthy and in the hands of skilled rowers quickly moves through the surf. Here father Tom McLaughlin rows with his son out through the surf.
Courtesy of Dave Pearson.

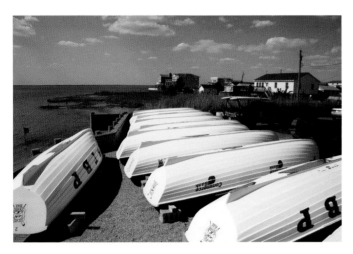

A fleet of Van Duynes at Long Beach Township lie in wait for the start of the summer season. As the largest lifeguard crew in New Jersey, they have forty-two surfboats. Some of the boats are sponsored by local businesses giving them advertising exposure to thousands of beachgoers.

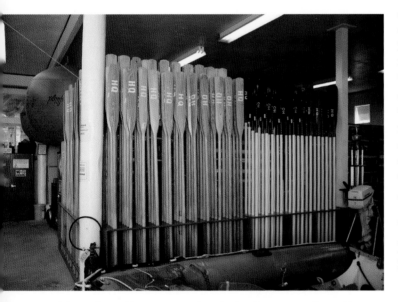

A large fleet of boats require hundreds of oars as evidenced by just part of the massive collection at Long Beach Township.

Since 1951, the Van Duyne Boat Works of Linwood have been constructing fiberglass skiffs that have similarities to the Hankins, but handle quite differently in the surf. Today, there are hundreds of these skiffs in service throughout eastern United States from Maine to Florida, including the Jersey Shore.

The Hankins boat had a third set of rowlocks for standup rowing, very popular in Monmouth County. The bottom was also flatter making it more stable when it was being launched or landed. But, the 17'3" Van Duyne had watertight compartments, making it virtually unsinkable — and that was an excellent selling point.

Shortly before Charles Hankins' death on June 24, 2003, Bobby Asay, formerly of Asbury Park and now residing in Florida, had begun to put his woodworking

skills to work and produced boats that were lighter and faster than both Van Duyne and Hankins. In later years, he used the wood prototype to create fiberglass skiffs that are now in use throughout Monmouth and Ocean County.

It is unlikely any more wooden skiffs will be constructed, as nearly all of the boat builders today use fiberglass. Competing against the Van Duyne is the Patroni, manufactured by Patroni Machine and Design out of Margate; they make a self-bailer, as well as the Schock Dory, another self-bailer manufactured in California. Other builders such as Warren Naus of Morganville, George R. Van Sant of Atlantic City, Robinson, Pharo Boat Works, and Bud Campbell of Neptune City constructed wooden skiffs, but never in sufficient volume to become classics.

Boats were launched right off the sand or off special rollers to make the job easier. Skilled crews launched themselves while additional handlers launched rookies and others who were just learning. They would wait for a lull in the waves and push off shore. If they timed it right and kept moving forward with the bow pointed into the waves, they would make it past the surf zone in thirty seconds or so. If the timing was off, they popped an oar losing their forward momentum or somehow got turned sideways, they risked taking a wave over the side, flooding the boat and washing it to shore. The worst case in the boat is "going over the falls." This happened when the wave caught the boat stalled in the water and washes it in backwards, inevitably resulting in capsizing and perhaps even injury to the rower.

Competitive rowing events are as old as the lifeguard boats themselves. Winning a big rowing event gave prestige and bragging rights to the crews who often train year round for the events.

Development of the Rescue Flotation Device (RFD)

When lifeguards make a rescue, they swim to the victim with some type of flotation device. This eliminates direct contact with the victim and gives them something to hold on to and float. The earliest of these was the standard rescue ring or ring buoy. It could best be described as a floating donut with ropes attached to the outer circumference. The rescuer would sling a rope loop over their shoulder and swim to the victim and tow them to shore.

In Ship Bottom prior to 1929, life rings were the main apparatus used to rescue victims. Purchase of the life rings came as a result of local residents taking up a collection, asking each resident for a ten-cent donation. The circular buoy was not streamlined, so lifeguard crews looked for something better.

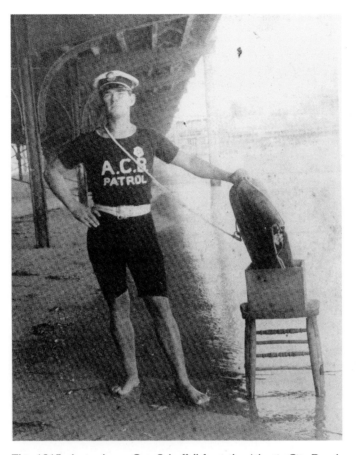

This 1915 photo shows Guy Schaffell from the Atlantic City Beach Patrol with a diamond rescue can in front of the Brighton Casino. Note the sling to attach the rescue device to the rescuer. *Alfred M. Heston Collection – Atlantic City Free Public Library.*

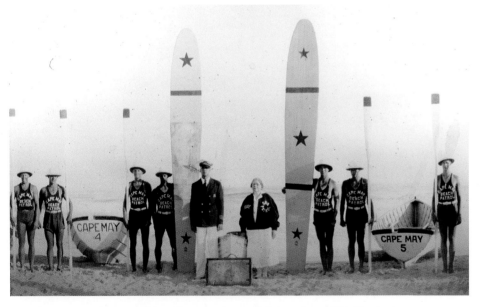

Cape May Beach Patrol used these fourteen-foot paddleboards in 1937. The Ocean City Beach Patrol was the first to use them as rescue gear in 1934. The first board was purchased from Hawaiian surfboard champion Tom Blake. *Courtesy of Buzz Mogck, Cape May Beach Patrol.*

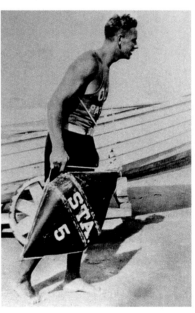

Ocean City Lifeguard William Young is pictured with a diamond rescue can in 1920. The canvas covered rescue device was lighter and safer than the metal cans and ropes attached to the perimeter allowed the victim to grab a hold. *Courtesy of Fred Miller.*

The answer was in torpedo shaped metal rescue cans. Developed by Captain Henry Sheffield in 1897, they were buoyant and streamlined. Sharply pointed at both ends, they were constructed from sheet metal, and had lines stretched along the outside. Invariably they were painted red. Although an improvement over the ring buoy, the construction presented its own hazards. The sharp points made them potentially deadly aquatic missiles and although it may be merely a beach legend, reportedly, because of their metal construction, they attracted lightning!

In 1901, the Atlantic City lifeguards announced a new buoy constructed of copper that was diamond shaped and capable of supporting five men. Ocean City lifeguards contended it was too cumbersome and proceeded with their own materials and designs. Captain

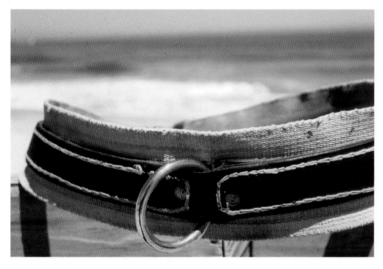

The canvas and leather belt with a brass ring at the back was standard lifeguard issue for decades. The rescue device was clipped to the ring to be swum out to the victim.

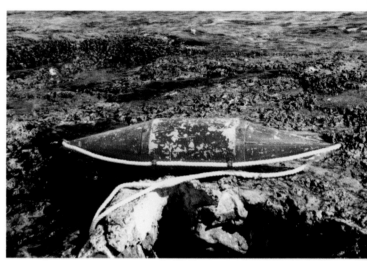

The pointed ends of the hollow metal buoy made it a dangerous projectile. It reportedly was also a target for lightning. Improvements were made shortly thereafter. *Courtesy of Charles Hartl.*

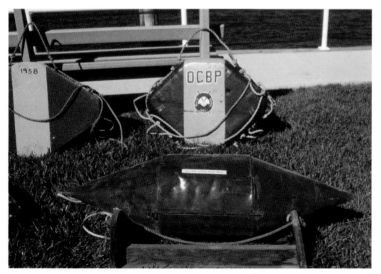

The metal rescue can (foreground) replaced the ring buoy. Pointy ends placed anyone in its way at risk. The diamond cans pictured were an improvement.

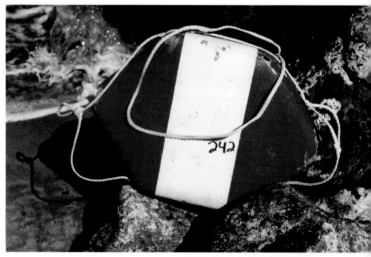

Foam covered with fiberglass buoys replaced the metal rescue cans. They were prone to cracking and splitting but provided good buoyancy. *Courtesy of Charles Hartl.*

Jack Jernee of the Ocean City Beach Patrol in 1922 developed a type of diamond can that was "simple in construction, easy to operate, practically indestructible and approved after the most severe of tests."

Local companies, including A & P Supermarkets, began to manufacture diamond and torpedo shaped rescue cans. They were manufactured from several materials including aluminum, balsa wood, and foam. The design known as the diamond can won out and became the standard lifesaving device.

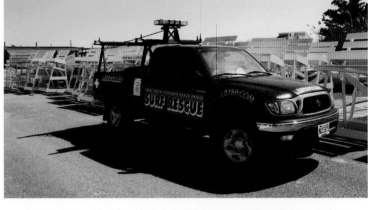

Rescue trucks enable lifeguards from New Jersey's largest lifeguard crew, Long Beach Township, to quickly respond to emergencies along their twelve miles of beach.

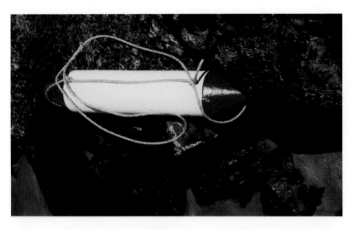

Balsa wood buoys covered with canvas were the next generation of lifesaving devices. It was strung with ropes to allow the victim to grasp it. *Courtesy of Charles Hartl.*

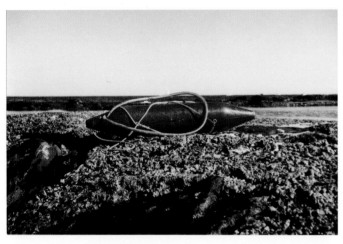

The precursor to modern molded buoys was constructed from fiberglass. *Courtesy of Charles Hartl.*

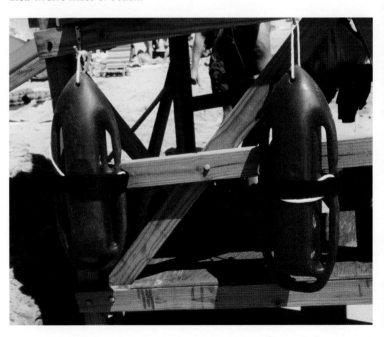

Injection molded rescue cans with integrated handles and slings comprise modern rescue gear.

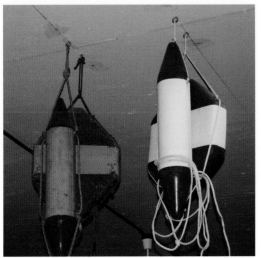

Two generations of rescue cans hang in lifeguard headquarters at Long Beach Township.

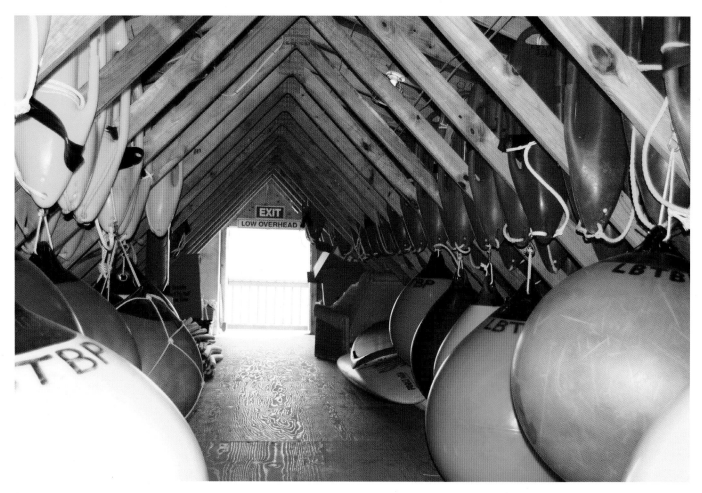

Winter storage of the over four hundred rescue cans maintained by the Long Beach Township Beach Patrol. Their inventory is massive and this photo captures just a small portion of their rescue gear.

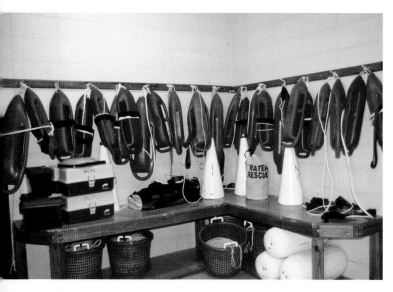

Crews keep an ample supply of rescue cans.

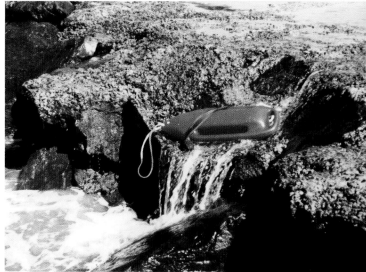

The classic Burnside Rescue can — sold and distributed by Marine Rescue Products in Rhode Island — are the staple of lifeguard crews throughout the world. Hundreds of thousands are in service. *Courtesy of Charles Hartl.*

In 1968, Lieutenant Bob Burnside of Los Angeles County revolutionized the design of the rescue buoy with what has become the standard throughout the world. He imagined that it might be made of plastic, consulted with an industrial design expert in a new process known as rotational plastic molding, and the Burnside buoy was born. This iconic rescue device, much copied, now allows lifeguards to rescue multiple victims without worry that the device will injure them or their rescuers.

Rescue Reels and Line Buckets

New Jersey lifeguards depend on rescue lines to rapidly bring in victims caught in rip currents. For many years, the lines were wound on rescue reels that were set in front of the lifeguard stand. Guards would "hook up" to the line with a clip that attached to their rescue belts. Running into the surf caused the reel to spin at high speed; if there wasn't a second guard to slow down the spin, it would result in a backlash, fouling the line, and making it ineffective.

In later years, a simple solution was found in line buckets. Line is stacked in an open bucket, very much like the faking boxes used by the United States Life-Saving Service. No matter how fast the line is run out, it will never foul since it has no moving parts. The standard length is six hundred feet. A guard on a line and RFD rescue is attached to shore based line pullers, just about guaranteeing their rapid return to shore. It is extraordinarily effective in retrieving multiple victims caught in rip currents. In some cases as many as six victims at a time can be brought to shore, a feat that would be just about impossible without the line!

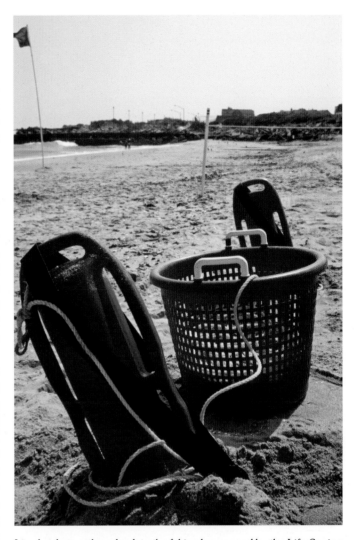

Line buckets, a throwback to the faking boxes used by the Life-Saving Service have replaced spools which invariably backlashed after guards running to a rescue caused them to spin at high speed. Here, Adolph Keifer Rescue Cans are attached to a 600-foot rescue line.

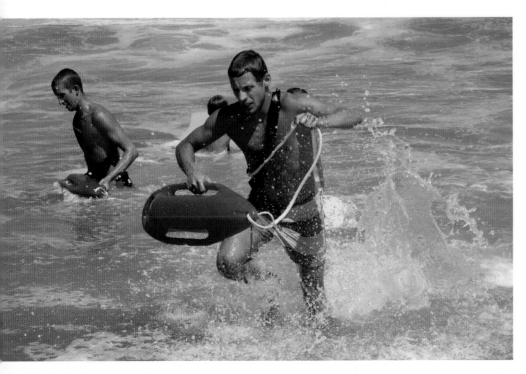

A rescue can from Marine Rescue Products is shown in action during an actual rescue.
Courtesy of Monmouth County Park System.

The efficiency of the rescue line translates into a grueling competitive event in lifeguard tournaments referred to as the "land line" event. Guards swim the line to a competitor "victim" who is rescued and pulled in by one, two, or three line pullers.

Early Lifeguard Equipment

Typical for Jersey Shore Patrol

Canvas and leather belt: The staple for decades was a lifeguard rescue belt that was designed to be worn loosely about the waist. It had a heavy canvas backing with a thick leather belt sewn to it. It had a standard belt buckle in the front and a brass ring to attach rescue devices in the back.

Metal Rescue Can: Called this because of their metal "can-like" construction and usually painted red, it was a barrel with two pointed ends. Lines attached to it enabled the rescuer to swim it out through the surf.

Diamond Rescue Can: Named for its shape, it was a marked improvement over the metal cans. Constructed from a canvas or fiberglass covering over balsa wood or cork, it too had lines attached for the victim to grasp and the lifeguard to tow.

Rescue Reel: This was simply a horizontal roller of rescue line mounted on a box or metal stand. The guard would attach the line directly to himself or to the rescue can. Onshore line pullers would quickly retrieve both rescuer and victim. Most reels have been abandoned because they easily backlash, opting for the more effective line buckets, similar to the faking boxes used by the Life-Saving Service.

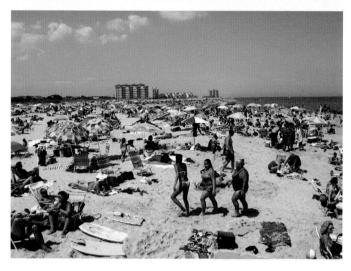

Holidays bring massive crowds to beachfronts such as this busy weekend day at Joline Avenue Beach at Seven Presidents Oceanfront Park in Long Branch. Author Ted Olsen is beach captain here.

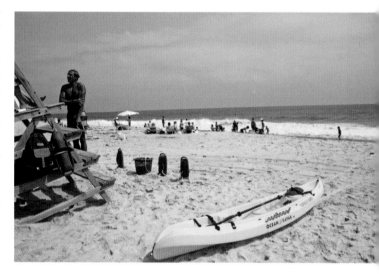

Kayaks have become a preferred rescue and patrol device. Faster, lighter, easier to maintain, and less expensive than surfboats, they can navigate heavy surf with an experienced paddler. Many crews have "fleets" of these versatile boats.

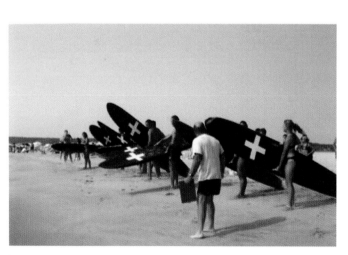

Surfboards became "rescue boards" when they were brought from Hawaii to Long Beach California in 1913. They began to appear in New Jersey in the 1930s, and Howard Rowland claimed he brought them here. Lifeguards at Sandy Hook practice paddleboard rescues during a rookie training camp. *Courtesy of Dave Pearson.*

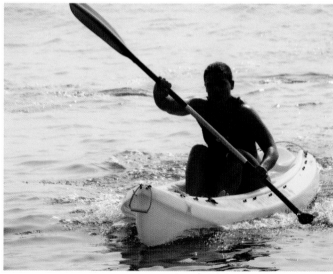

Kayaks can be easily handled by lifeguards, making them excellent for patrol. They are also a great conditioning device making them good for workouts. *Courtesy of Alice Kantor.*

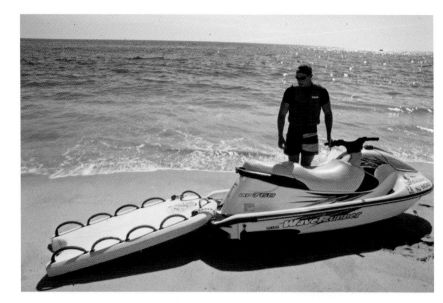

The latest generation of rescue craft is PWC's (Personal Water Craft). These high-speed, rescue devices towing rescue sleds are capable of reaching speeds approaching 60-mph and can quickly transport victims through dangerously rough surf. Although easy to use in a recreational context, a great deal of training is necessary to operate them as rescue crafts, especially in heavy seas, and New Jersey law requires rescue operators to have a boating safety certification issued from the State Police.

Long Beach Township Beach Patrol maintains a fleet of three Inflatable Rescue Boats or (IRBs). They have a rigid hull with an inflatable collar, powered by an outboard motor. Special teams are trained in their use and undergo rigorous rescue exercises. Each boat is equipped with radios, rescue tubes, lines and CPR masks. The program consists of six officers consisting of a coordinator and five drivers.
Courtesy of Long Beach Township Beach Patrol.

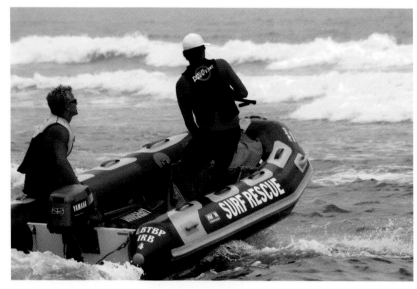

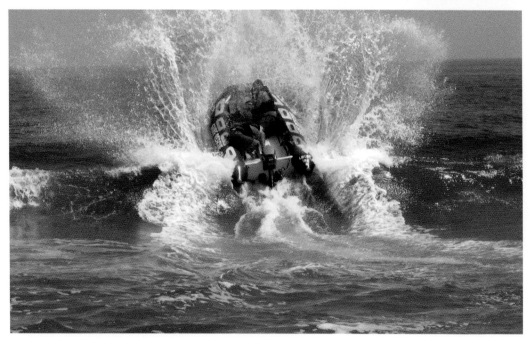

IRB's are used to deal with uncooperative beach patrons, often times surfers, windsurfers, and personal watercraft users. They can also be used to keep offshore boats from encroaching on bathing areas.
Courtesy of Long Beach Township Beach Patrol.

The Day I Almost Drowned

Michael "Spike" Fowler,
Lifeguard Supervisor
Monmouth County Park System

The surf was really "cranked" from a big nor'easter that had come in, but the weather had cleared and the rain had stopped. There were fifteen to twenty-five foot waves offshore and we were about to take a sixteen-foot surfboat into them. Nothing would back me off in those days so I stupidly agreed to row with the Crocker brothers, not realizing it would almost become my last day on earth.

I was to row the suicide seat a.k.a. the bow. Richie and I got behind the oars, and Kenny launched us into the heavy surf, just behind the protective "L" jetty by the Shark River Inlet. With Kenny riding in the back, we got offshore perhaps fifty yards or so and a huge wave rolled over the bow, immediately sinking us. However, we managed to wash back in. We dumped the boat and went back out. We made it out about the same distance — and another wave came over the bow with the same results. Should we try again? "Let's go," said the Crockers. So we were back out and, with sheer luck, made it out beyond the breakers.

A large crowd had gathered by now, not only to see us, but the Coast Guard offshore in their motorized lifeboat. With its watertight compartments, it was unsinkable, and if it rolled over, would right itself. They were conducting rough water drills. They were aghast we were there. We chatted with the crewmen for a bit who had donned heavy-duty life preservers and were tethered to their craft in case the boat went over. Of course, we didn't even have lifejackets on — we were lifeguards!

The waves were enormous and dwarfed our boat! I had never seen waves so big. All we had to do now was get back to shore and the only way we could do that was ride one of those monster waves in and I was absolutely scared. We had to look for a small wave and after sizing up the situation saw

one coming and started rowing to catch it. If you're too late, you'll miss the wave and if you're too early and too far in front of it — you're dead as the boat will career wildly out of control. So we rowed and tried to time it just right and, just as we thought we caught it, Richie dumped his oars as you're supposed to. But we didn't. We missed the wave. I had my oars and started backing out while Kenny jumped off the stern to recover the oars his brother dumped. We're backing out, backing out, when the largest wave I've ever seen formed just off the stern. We were trapped inside the surf zone! I dumped my oars and grabbed the sides of the boat and held on for my life. The wave seemed twice the height of the length of the boat. We went halfway up the wave and the stern came over the top of me. I was plunged into darkness as the boat cart wheeled lengthwise!

We were all thrown clear and left a quarter-mile offshore in raging surf. The Crockers would stay with the boat; I would swim in and get help to recover the boat. As I started for shore, wave after wave pounded me and I was getting sucked out by the rip currents. I was embroiled in the highly aerated water making it difficult to keep my head above it, and every time I made it to the surface, another crushing wave came in on top driving me down. I was exhausted but could see that lifeguards on shore were coming to my rescue. I was drowning.

The guards never made it out to rescue me. It was too rough and they just kept getting washed back. Somehow, someway, with the last ounce of energy and determination, I managed to make it to shore. It took nine guards forty-five minutes to recover the Crockers and the boat, which almost smashed against the Lincoln Avenue jetty.

About ten years later I was at Campbell's Boatyard in Neptune City, talking with an old boat builder. He was the stereotypical old salt with tanned and leathered skin, wearing coveralls and suspenders. We started with our stories of bravado and he began to tell the tale of foolhardy lifeguards in Avon taking a boat out in raging surf and how he'd never seen such a sight as when that gigantic wave capsized their boat and, describing the day I almost drowned, he remarked: "I've never seen a bigger wave. One fellow almost drowned. The lifeguards couldn't even rescue him. Those guys are lucky to be alive."

Chapter Six
The Culture of Lifeguarding

Fun in the sun, wild women, and wild lifeguard parties...that's what it's all about. Critics think lifeguards don't work real jobs, like in construction. Get tan, listen to a radio, go swimming, meet people, ogle girls in bikinis — this is the image. The June 1980 issue of *Cosmopolitan* magazine cast the typical stereotype with their feature article "Those Lusty, Legendary, Lifeguards," asking its readers: "Have you every wondered what untamed passions lurk within the golden hero of your beach as he surveys the surf?"

This is part of the perceived "culture" of being a lifeguard.

However, it's not just a summer job — it's a lifestyle, say many seasoned lifeguard veterans. What begins as seasonal employment frequently turns into a lifetime vocation. This summer job becomes a way of life, and often full time employment is tailored to the lifeguard experience. Many lifeguards pursue careers in teaching in order to continue their calling to the beach, surf, sun, and all that goes along with it.

The past, negative image of lifeguarding becomes a public relations challenge for beach supervisors. There have been television advertisements portraying lifeguards in less than flattering roles, usually involving watching women, tanned as a result of the sponsor's product, and not watching the water. The feature motion picture "Lifeguard" chronicled the struggle of Sam Elliott (the star lifeguard) had between pursuing his love of working on the California beach versus pressure to obtain a "real" job — in this case as a salesman of expensive sports cars. Television shows like "Baywatch" heighten the drama faced by guards.

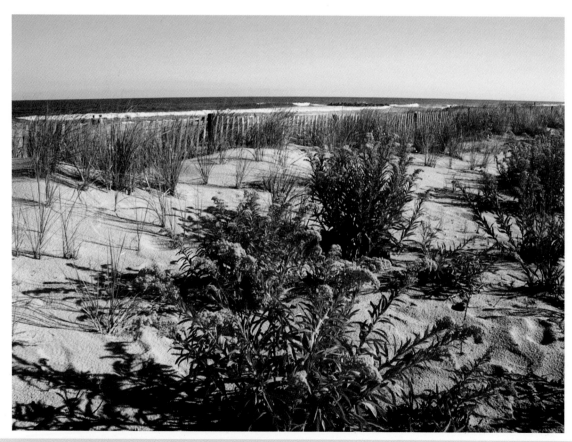

Fall brings beautiful color to the dunes along the Jersey Shore such as here in Belmar.

Overcoming these stereotypes exasperates most lifeguard leaders. "People just don't understand" is the prevalent attitude. The hours of training and conditioning every day, completing the numerous certifications, dangerous doses of sunlight contributing to pre-mature aging and skin cancer, cold weather and water, rain, lightning, jellyfish stings, and the risk they face entering rough water to rescue victims. Lifeguards have an obligation to attend work each day in order to safeguard the public. They do not have the luxury of taking random days off, calling out, or taking vacations. Job attendance is essential. Supervisors are uneasy in trusting the public's safety to young, inexperienced guards. In short, a lifeguard must report for work or risk jeopardizing his crew and the public. This explains why crews are balanced with senior personnel, regular lifeguards, and rookies.

Many professions have at least some cultural component whether they are police officers or coal miners — and lifeguards are no different. There are the "rookie rites of passage," with the goal of new guards to survive rookie year naiveté and move to the rank of experienced lifeguard. As a result, there are good-natured pranks invoked on fellow crewmembers. The book *All Summer Long*, by Gordon Hesse, "captures behind-the-scenes stories of beach culture as seen and told by lifeguards in their own words." Yes, the late night beer binges and sexual conquests are covered!

Lifeguards are not just a bunch of employees. They are a crew and a team with a sense of brotherhood. Teams compete fiercely for bragging rights and the job breeds lifetime friendships. Fathers and mothers pass their lifesaving legacy to sons and daughters and the shore is rife with multi-generation lifeguards.

There is no denying the job is fun and glamorous, but many people fail to see the component of responsibility. It is a profession where a 99.99 percent success rate is unacceptable. Lifeguards constantly make the difference between life and death. When the beach is crowded with thousands of people and it is a bright, hot, and sunny weekend and the surf is cranking with a northeast swell with rips everywhere, it becomes an awesome responsibility. When one hundred people dive under a wave — and only ninety-nine pop back up — the lifeguard has to spot this and respond. The challenge is awesome.

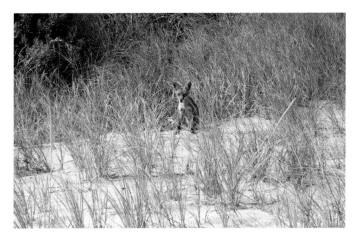

Humans are not the only species that enjoy the beach — as evidenced by this red fox in the dunes at Seven Presidents Oceanfront Park in Long Branch.

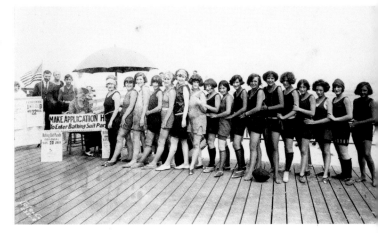

The Miss America Pageant got its start in 1921 in Atlantic City. It was originally billed as a beauty contest, but that was later changed to provide scholarships to young women. Several shore municipalities hosted their own beauty pageants and bathing suit parades such as this one in Bradley Beach in 1923. Bathing beauties are a staple in New Jersey beach culture. *Courtesy of Dick Johnson.*

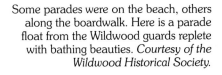

Some parades were on the beach, others along the boardwalk. Here is a parade float from the Wildwood guards replete with bathing beauties. *Courtesy of the Wildwood Historical Society.*

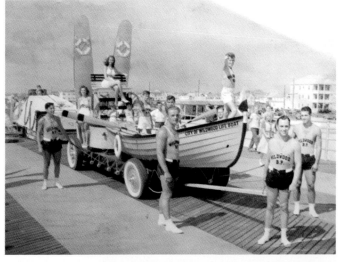

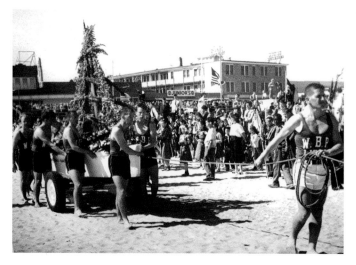

Some lifeguard crews would participate in elaborate preseason celebrations as shown in Wildwood where they would drive flowers into the ocean to commemorate Memorial Day.
Courtesy of the Wildwood Historical Society.

The Rites of Passage, Rituals, and Pranks

~ A rookie, tired of his lunch being eaten every day by senior guards, laced his cookies with a strong laxative. The problem was solved.

~ Rookies are sent searching for twenty-five feet of shoreline, keys to the oarlocks, jetty wrenches, and jetty stretchers. They are always just one beach away.

~ Whistle tests. Rookies are sent to the end of the jetty to test their whistle volume with the directive that senior guards will wave to them when they hear the signal. They never wave while the rookie blows his brains out for the entire beach to hear.

~ Lifeguards will occasionally swallow small, live, baitfish for the shock value. George Herbert of Avon once consumed thirteen wriggling fish after I (author Fowler) had quit at nine.

~ Rookies are instructed to come back with names, ages, and availability status of attractive ladies, paving the way for senior guards.

~ Most everyone gets a nickname of sorts. Crackers, the Riddler, Captain Cruel, Mick, Krusty, Frog, Harp, the Cheese Brothers, and Frankie Goombah have all worked our local beaches. Tattoos are also very popular.

~ By the end of rookie season, they will have done thousands of pushups, sit-ups, pull-ups, swims, and runs. Rookies may find remnants of sea life in their bags such as dead fish or live crabs.

~ Some guards are bottomless eating machines. Rookies are instructed to come back with food. "We don't care where you get it, but come back with food." Interestingly, often patrons contribute to their quest.

~ Stand "Baseball" is played by young virile, male lifeguards. As attractive females pass by the stand, guards will try to get a hit by waving. If she waves back, it's a single. If the guard can get the girl to wave back while holding hands with her boyfriend, it's a home run.

~ Though not happening in today's society, rookies of years ago could have their bathing suits removed by a gang of senior guards. The only solution was to run in the ocean where they were likely to be left a long time until a kind colleague swam out a suit.

~ Boat wars and stand wars sometimes break out on slow summer days. One beach will attack and sink the other's boat, leaving them to struggle getting back to shore. One beach spread honey beneath the other's stand attracting swarms of bugs. One crew of midnight lifeguard raiders completely buried their rival's boat and stand. One morbid prank involved the nailing of a spread-eagled raccoon road kill to the seat of their rival's stand.

In Their Own Words: Lifeguards Share Stories

Meeting Joe of the Asbury Park Lifeguards
Harry Hoehn, Lifeguard Veteran

The first time I walked into there, it was their end of the year event in 1990. The first thing Joe did was hand me a bottle of beer, then say "hello." He poured down his bottle of beer, took it and smashed it against the wall in the lifeguard room. Then he took another one, took one sip and smashed the whole thing against the wall. That was my introduction to Joe.

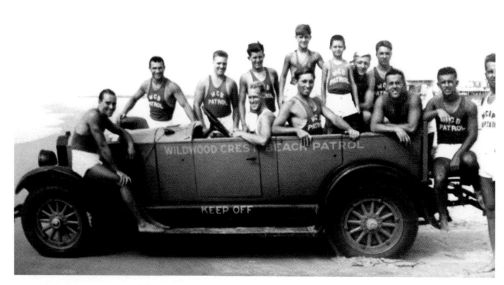

The fellowship seems evident in this 1930 picture of Wildwood Beach Patrol.
Courtesy of the Wildwood Historical Society.

"*Wanna Be*" *Lifeguards*
Don Myers, Lifeguard Chief
Long Beach Township

Commenting on the difficulty of the test, the athleticism, and training required for the job: a lot of these "wanna be" lifeguards are just down for the "3 S's": sun, suds, and sex.

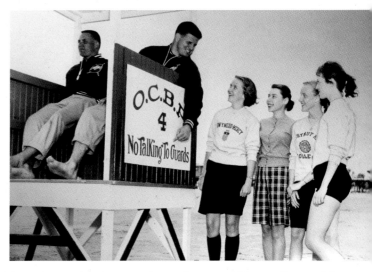

According to the sign, people are discouraged from talking to lifeguards in Ocean City. That does not seem to faze these admiring females. *Courtesy of Fred Miller.*

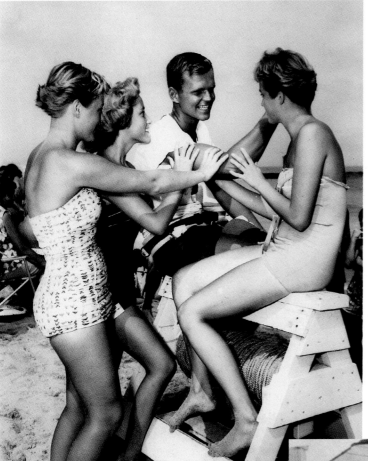

The attraction of young ladies to tanned and athletic lifeguards is inevitable. This staged press photo taken in the 1950s features Avon-by-the-Sea lifeguard Joseph Jasaitis who became a renowned Jersey Shore physician.
Courtesy of Joseph Jasaitis.

Wildwood Lifeguards pose on the boardwalk opposite the theater showing the 1970 movie "Lifeguard," starring Sam Elliott. Note the inviting tag line "Every girl's summer dream"! The movie profoundly influenced public perception of lifeguards. *Courtesy of the Wildwood Historical Society.*

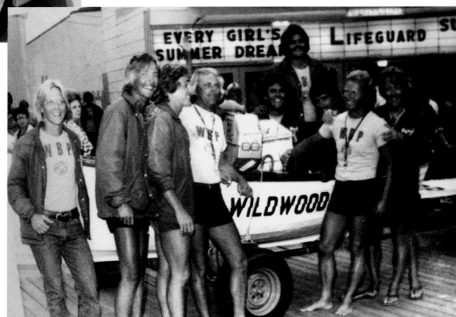

What it Takes to be a Rookie Lifeguard
Andrew Fedick, Rookie of the Year 2008
Monmouth County Park System

What better summer job is there than that of a lifeguard? I would get to work every day in the sun, on a beach, and get a great tan. I thought I had an idea of what the job entailed. I had seen lifeguards on the job every summer at various beaches. They kept an eye on the water, blew their whistle at some rowdy teenagers chicken-fighting in the water, jogged on the boardwalk, practiced a few rescue drills, and once in a while went on a real rescue.

When I read about tryouts for lifeguarding at Seven Presidents Oceanfront Park for the Monmouth County Park System, a beach I had never been to but was close to my university, I jumped right on it. I quickly learned I was horribly mistaken as to what the job really entails. Not only was there a rigorous set of tests to pass against about a dozen other highly qualified competitors all looking to

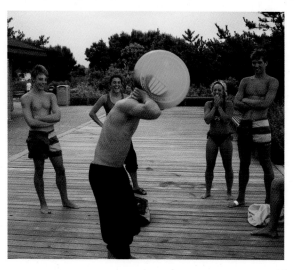

There always seems to be some time for fooling around.

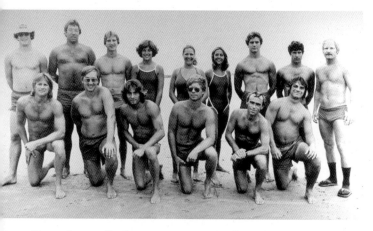

Team photos offer the opportunity to sneak in pranks...here lifeguard Bill Wishart wears black socks with sandals. Author Michael Fowler is in the front row, fourth from left. *Courtesy of Susan Rosenberg.*

fill the same position as I was, but every day on the job was as demanding as the next. My lifeguard supervisor said on my first day that I would end the summer in the best shape of my life. He was not exaggerating. Each day was a physical challenge. Every morning started with an arduous beach workout, followed by hard physical activity throughout the remainder of the day. I had never met a group of people so passionate and intense about physical fitness. This lifeguarding crew was like none I had ever seen. I thought I was already in great shape going into my first day of work.... I puked after my first lifeguard workout. I guess not.

As a rookie lifeguard, each day is a tryout, and I was under the constant watch of my supervisor, captains, and lieutenants. I was drilled the hardest, was the first man in the water on rescues to gain experience, and had the most to learn from radio 10-codes, rescue protocol, how to properly set up our life-saving equipment, and even how to recognize patterns in weather, winds, tides and rip-currents. Most importantly, I quickly learned how tight-knit the lifeguard crew was. It made perfect sense after realizing how much we need to depend on each other for both our safety and the safety of our patrons. I can say I am in the best shape of my life after this past summer, and cannot wait for June to come again.

"I Did Exactly What You Asked Me to Do"
Michael "Spike" Fowler, Lifeguard Supervisor
Monmouth County Park System

Bobby Morris was a rookie in Avon in 1982 and his adversary was Elliot Cohen, an experienced veteran lifeguard. It's now Dr. Elliot Cohen I might add.

Rookie initiations were quite the "in thing" in the 1980s. This was aside from the physical torment — the constant swims, runs, practice rescues, pushups and even requirements to swallow whole live fish that had been seined out of the cove. Anyway, Bobby came to me on several occasions to complain that Elliot kept bothering him. At first I dismissed his complaints as simple trials and tribulations of the job and lifeguarding culture, but they began to escalate. Bobby was now coming to me greatly distressed. "Mr. Fowler — Elliot's bothering me again." So I spoke to Elliot and instructed him to leave him alone. Bobby came to me again, more distressed. I demanded of Elliot to leave him alone.

Things were better for a week or so, but finally Bobby appeared before me once more, choking back tears of desperation. That was it. I tracked down Elliot and gave him his last warning or else — "Leave Bobby Morris alone!"

Finally it was over. Summer was moving along just fine now, or so I thought. Elliot and Bobby seemed to be getting along just fine — no complaints and I was happy when I watched the two of them take out the surfboat for a row to the buoy and back. I watched carefully as they rowed offshore, convinced they were now just about best friends — they were rowing as a team. My calm turned to concern, however, when Elliot came back in by himself. Bobby was missing.

When they got to the bell buoy, about a half-mile off Shark River Inlet, Elliot told Bobby that all lifeguards climb up the buoy and dive off. It was a rite of passage. This buoy had a huge bell on it that could be heard for at least a mile. Elliot climbed up first while Bobby steadied the boat, and deftly dove off. "Your turn!" exclaimed Elliot. As Bobby climbed the buoy tower, Elliot calmly rowed away.

So when Elliot landed solo, I immediately and excitedly asked where Bobby was. "He's at the buoy," said Elliot. I flew into a rage and when all was said and done, Elliot turned to me and in a soft voice said, "I did exactly what you asked me to do. You told me to 'leave him alone' — I left him alone."

My assistant Howie Hardie and I had to launch a rescue mission. When we arrived at the buoy, Bobby was all "gonged out." The bell's tolling had gotten to him and as he climbed into the stern of the boat for the ten-minute row to shore, he said hardly a word. He appeared as a rag doll. You could tell in his face that again he was fighting tears — he was a broken rookie.

At the time I was furious with both Elliot and Bobby over the whole incident, but God has a way of making you forget Bobby's misfortune and Elliot's deception. I cannot recall the story today without laughing out loud — and I've told this story many, many times.

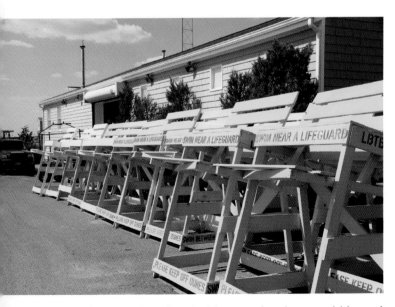

At Long Beach Township, freshly painted and prepared lifeguard stands wait, just as lifeguards do, in anticipation of the busy upcoming summer season.

Lifeguarding in Belmar in 1942
Anecdote by Bob Watkins, age 85
Belmar Lifeguard 1941 – 1947

We worked from 8 a.m. to 5 p.m. and had to clean the beach. They gave us potato sacks and had two rules for cleaning. No "heel and toe" — you couldn't use your feet to bury trash — you had to pick it up. The second was "no airplanes." Guards would take newspaper trash and let it fly downwind so the guys on the next beach would have to pick it up.

Rookie pay was $22.50 per week and second year guards made $25.00 per week. We would have all done it for nothing. That's how great the job was.

In 1944, they had girls in Belmar (because of the shortage of men due to the war effort). There was Doris Pflug and Jennie Bonk.

I had a trick for the team photos. I would build a sand mountain to stand on so I would look taller 'cause I'm short and I pulled out the shoulder straps on my tank top to make my shoulders look wider. It worked.

Looking at the team photos from the 1940s in May 2009 — "They're all dead. I'm the only one still alive. I've outlived them all."

Which is More Difficult?
Michael "Spike" Fowler,
Lifeguard Supervisor and College Professor

Another guard once asked me, "Which is the more challenging job, being a college professor or a lifeguard?"

I asked if a college professor had a ninety-nine percent mastery of the subject, would that be impressive? He responded, "Of course, it would be excellent!"

I then asked if a lifeguard had a ninety-nine percent success rate, would that be impressive?

The point was made.

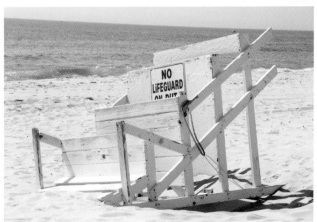

A lone lifeguard stand, left on the beach on sunny spring day in Spring Lake, awaits a summer revival.

Chapter Seven
Lifeguard Legends and Heroes

Colorful characters emerged through the years and lifeguards became legends. These figures are rich in culture and stories about them span generations. As stories are told, the truth gets stretched somewhat. But they are the mainstay of lifeguard events and veterans love to tell tales. These are stories of some of the great men who lifeguarded our New Jersey beaches.

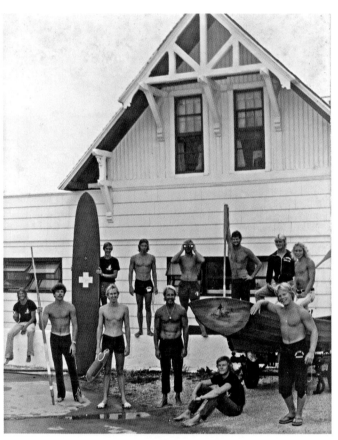

With the lifesaving station as a backdrop, the Takanassee lifeguards are pictured circa 1974. Shore area lifeguard legend Dick Martin is pictured in the center with his arms at his side and national swimming champion John Skinner is pictured in the surfboat holding the oar. Skinner was an Olympics contender but was not eligible to represent the U.S. because he was from South Africa. *Courtesy of Beth Woolley.*

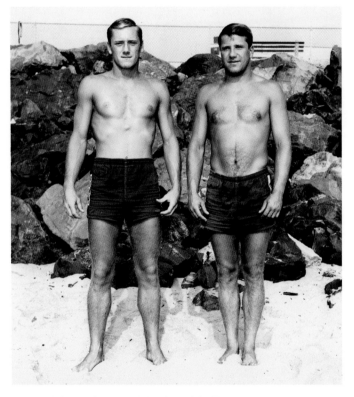

Veteran lifeguard Michael "Mick" Fidek (R) won numerous rowing championships during his long career as an Asbury Park lifeguard. Here he is in 1965 with Philip Huhn (L), who went on to become mayor of Long Branch. *Courtesy of McLaughlin Magazine.*

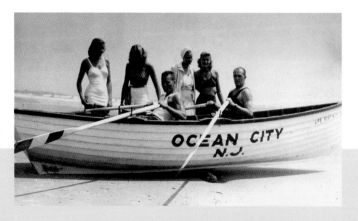

The famous Kelly Family from Philadelphia summered in Ocean City. Seated at the bow oars is John B. and at the stern is his son Jack, Jr. Second from left in the back row is Grace Kelly who became Princess Grace from Monaco as well as an American film star. John and Jack are the only father-son persons in the Ocean City Hall of Fame. The photo was taken August 9, 1947. *Courtesy of Fred Miller.*

Howard Rowland,
August 23, 1907 – February 22, 1988

Certainly one of the shore's most endearing lifesavers was Howard Rowland. Although he was not particularly tall, he was a giant of a man. In both physical size around his chest and in deed he was a giant. He could strike fear into the most seasoned lifeguard when time came for him to test your "skills." Especially beloved by the Belmar Beach Patrol, they host an annual tournament in his honor titled the "Howard Rowland Memorial Lifeguard Tournament."

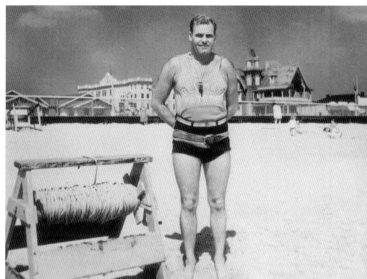

Howard Rowland on the beach in Belmar, 1959.

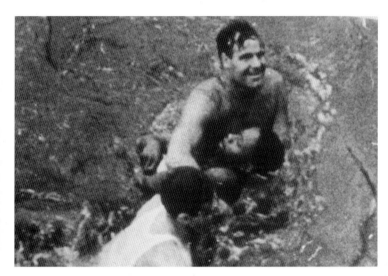

Born in Providence, Rhode Island, Howard Rowland's regular occupation was a fireman with the Asbury Park Fire Department. His list of accomplishments could span multiple pages, but highlights are that his first rescue was in 1918 at age 12, when he pulled a young girl out of Deal Lake. He is pictured here rescuing a child in Deal Lake circa 1950.

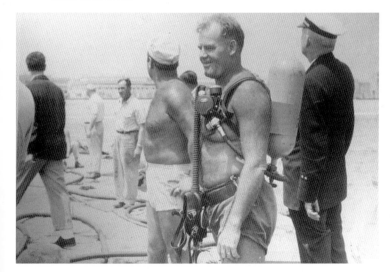

Rowland was also a water safety and first aid instructor. For thirty-five years, he chaired the Red Cross water safety program. One of the first rescuers to reach the wreck of the *Morro Castle,* he has been honored with dozens of citations. Allegedly he once rescued nineteen people in a single outing. Howard even delivered sixty-five babies. One of the pioneers of scuba diving, he is pictured here working on a body recovery at the 4th Avenue jetty in Asbury Park in 1947.

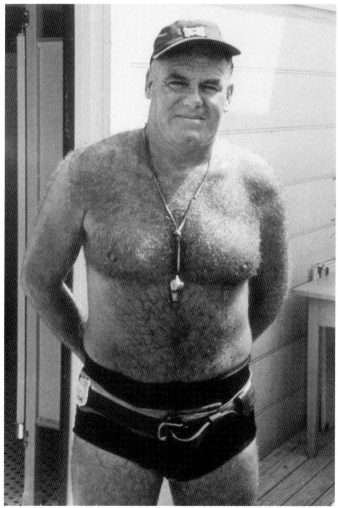

Rowland would pick the nastiest, roughest days, when the surf boiled with rip currents, huge waves, and storm conditions to test the guards. Striding down the beach with his blue Churchill fins, he struck terror into everyone, especially rookies who had been prompted via the many stories from the veterans. He is pictured here at his post in Belmar in 1957.

Of the many lifeguards interviewed that had to conduct a practice rescue of Rowland, the common thread was "respect and fear." Respect for perhaps the most skilled lifesaver to ever grace the shoreline, and fear for what he could do in the water to the rescuer. His barrel-like chest, which the lifeguard had to span to affect the rescue, was an impediment to begin with, but he always covered his body head to toe with copious amounts of tanning oil to make the job tougher. Howard took great pride and glee in his ability to take anyone under at anytime, and it always gave him the upper hand. When asked why he would do such a thing, he casually commented, "Just to see if they let go."

He had a comical side, often dressing up in a woman's bathing cap, demurely saying, "Help me Mr. Lifeguard! I can't swim!" He would then pounce on the rescuer and take him or her under. Sometimes he would dive beneath the surface just as the lifeguard approached. He would then circle up behind the rescuer, grab the line, and reel the guard down below the surface.

Several generations of lifeguards, particularly in Monmouth County, owe their lifesaving skills to this dedicated man who will live for a long time in the hearts of veteran lifesavers.

RIPLEY'S BELIEVE IT OR NOT!

HELP!

HOWARD ROWLAND, WHO BECAME HEAD LIFEGUARD OF THE BELMAR, N.J., BEACHES IN 1940, WAS STILL AT IT IN 1980 AT THE AGE OF 74. DURING HIS CAREER HE SAVED SOME 10,000 LIVES

© 1989 King Features Syndicate, Inc. World rights reserved   6-2.

One of the pioneers of modern lifeguarding, Howard was born in August, 1907 and died in February, 1988. He went on to become the world's oldest lifeguard. At his post daily, he supervised the lifeguards in Belmar up until age eighty working there for fifty years. The 10,000 is considered a bit of exaggeration — the real number being about 6,000.

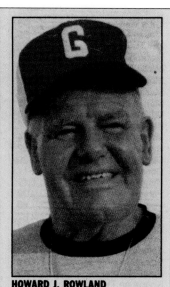

Rowland mastered the sea

By JO ANN MOSLOCK
Press Staff Writer

The mere memory still makes Tim Gallagher's face twist.

It's the summer of 1969 and Howard Rowland is striding along the surf in Avon, his silver whistle bobbing from his neck and his hairy chest slathered with baby oil. He stabs the air with a stubby forefinger toward the men perched in the lifeguard stand. Gallagher is one of them.

HOWARD J. ROWLAND
Friends recall him with respect

Rowland's passing in 1988 brought heartfelt praise throughout the lifeguard community with some referring to him as the "Patriarch of Lifeguarding." *Courtesy of Asbury Park Press.*

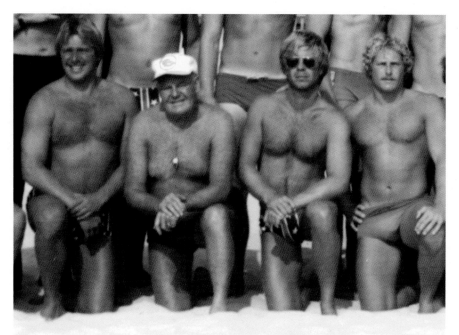

Lifeguard legend Howard Rowland in white cap. Author Michael Fowler is to his left. Rowland personally selected the stars and strips bathing suit motif for the 1976 Bicentennial celebration. Many guards objected to the small "cut" of the suit and put shells or outer suits over it.

Don Myers
Interviewed April 24, 2009

Imagine the responsibility of managing the largest lifeguard crew in New Jersey with 213 lifeguards manning fifty-four lifeguard stands along twelve miles of beach! Aside from the management of personnel, try keeping track of nine emergency response trucks, four inflatable rescue boats (IRBs), forty-two lifeguard boats, 236 paddleboards, and 412 rescue cans. Such is the job of lifeguard veteran Don Myers, lifeguard supervisor of the Long Beach Township Beach Patrol. Placed in another perspective, Don manages just a fraction short of ten percent of the 127 miles of shoreline between Sandy Hook and Cape May. His job is huge and he does it well.

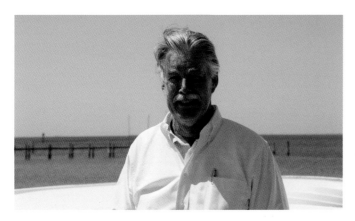

Head of the largest lifeguard crew in New Jersey, Don Myers oversees the operations of Long Beach Township Beach Patrol. His office overlooks the Bay.

Don is a 43-year veteran ocean lifeguard who began his career in 1967 at the age of eighteen. That was the minimum age lifeguards were hired then. He rose through the ranks and was appointed Assistant Captain in 1979 and to his present position in 1986.

Philosophic, articulate, and incredibly ambitious, Don maintains mountains of data in a maniacally organized fashion. Though modest (he gives the credit to his crew), he is particularly proud of the LIT or Lifeguard in Training program he pioneered. This program offers young, aspiring lifeguards, ages 11 through 15 the chance to train and become fit rescuers. It is also his primary feeder program to support his massive crew.

His office, with a comfortable sofa and yacht chairs overlooking the bay, replete with much wall memorabilia and an extensive library, reveals his commitment to total professionalism in lifeguarding. Don is well known and respected throughout the lifeguard community and certainly deserves a place among the "greats"!

Harry "Buzz" Mogck
Interviewed July 2, 2009

Buzz Mogck is chief officer of the Cape May City Beach Patrol. He received his nickname "Buzz" from his aunt at the age of two because he was very active as a child — buzzing all around. His rookie year was in 1967. Harry became a lifeguard because his father, who owned a local marina, sold the family business during his enlistment in the Army. Consequently, Harry returned home without any summer employment. At first, he was reluctant because he hadn't kept up with his swimming and fitness in two and half years. Fortunately for Harry, his luck and skill not only propelled him to pass the swim test, but also landed him a summer job for the next forty-three years.

In 1981, the captain's position became available. By now, his children were fairly grown and he had the experience for this new position. To Buzz, this became a golden opportunity because these positions are typically filled for one's lifetime.

Just a few years after receiving this position, Buzz would end up leading one of the greatest rescues ever performed in the beach patrol's history. In 1983, a Navy helicopter was flying a routine mission along the coast when it crashed just a mile off the beach. There were seven service men onboard. Approximately 25-30 Cape May lifeguards were involved in this gallant rescue. All service men were saved except for one member who was killed on impact. This unfortunate situation marked one of the proudest days of his career as his lifeguards demonstrated tremendous heroism and bravery for saving would-be victims from a sunken helicopter.

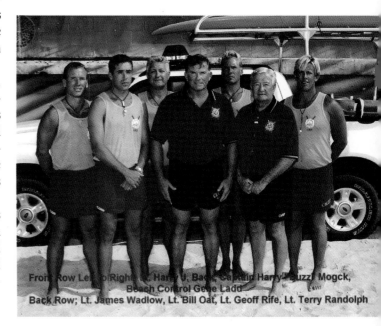

Cape May Beach Patrol officers in 2002: veteran Harry "Buzz" Mogck is pictured front row, center. *Courtesy of Buzz Mogck.*

Since this time, Buzz has remained at the captain's helm ready and willing to lead yet another daring and life-threatening rescue. He has been a major catalyst in advancing the lifeguarding profession in New Jersey. This includes: certifications, equipment upgrades, and technology to name just a few. When asked to reflect on Cape May Beach Patrol's greatest legacy, there is only one thing that comes to his mind. The pride he has that this crew both past and present has never had a single drowning on a guarded beach since its establishment in 1911.

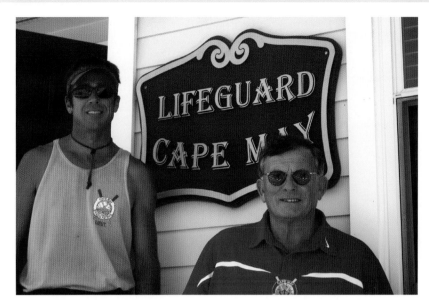

Veteran Cape May Beach Patrol lifeguard Harry "Buzz" Mogck (rt.) is at his headquarters with Lieutenant Harry Back.

Jack Schellenger
Interviewed February 14, 2006

Jack Schellenger came from a family of lifeguards including his uncle who in 1918 became Captain of the Beach Patrol in Cape May. His cousins were lifeguards and his father started in Cape May and became head of the guards in Point Pleasant Beach at Jenkinson's Pavilion. Jack started in 1955 when they gave him a whistle and beach assignment. He received no formal training — only on the job training. According to Jack, "If you lived in Cape May and you weren't a lifeguard, nobody knew you. It was just part of growing up in Cape May. And here I am fifty years later doing the same stuff."

After serving forty years in Cape May, he moved north to Wildwood where he was not only a lifeguard, but also an EMT/medic. He, as many long term lifeguards, went into education and was a teacher in the Freehold Regional School District as well as a basketball coach at several area schools. He is also a life member of the Freehold First Aid Squad. According to Cape May Beach Patrol Lieutenant Jim Wadlow, "He's dedicated his life to lifesaving."

Asked about memorable rescues, Jack recalled, "We had some boats that washed in and the lifeguards got involved with that. No sharks — knock on wood! I've seen sharks near guys fishing and they are not that far out unfortunately. The old history that they are not there — I can't believe that because that's their home. But they only come in if they are sick or hungry and that's very, very rare."

Jack's philosophy of lifeguarding is "prevention."

"I guess you can put it all together in one word. Prevent problems before they happen. Keep people out of the rips, undertows, keep them in close, not herded like cattle but you want to keep them in close and if you see the rips coming use the whistle to get them out of the rips."

Commenting on the use of lifeguard boats, Jack reminisces, "I think back to when I first started. They were wooden — they weighed, God knows, five or six hundred pounds and you were lucky if they floated. No one knew how to make fiberglass boats at that time."

Jack laughs heartily when talking about the old uniforms. "In Cape May and most south Jersey communities they wore wool shirts and when they got wet they itched like the devil. And then you got a pair of duck back pants or canvas pants and once they got wet they stayed wet and they would cause problems. And a jacket. That was about it. When those jackets got wet from the rain or whatever, the smell was atrocious. And today's uniform, the quick drying stuff and each patrol has their own rules and regulations when they have to wear shirts and when they don't." *(Author's note: Cape May Beach Patrol still requires guards to wear shirts whenever they are off the lifeguard stand.)*

Jack Schellenger, who continues to lifeguard to this day for the Wildwood Beach Patrol, says, "As long as my health holds out, I don't see an end anytime soon down the road."

My First Rescue
Jack Schellenger
Cape May Beach Patrol

I don't think I was on the beach more than an hour and a half my first day and it wasn't one of the nicest days of the year. There were a few bathers, a few swimmers … all of a sudden there was a middle-aged couple and my partner said they are going to get into trouble. I asked, "What do you mean?" He said, "Look at this rip current" or as we used to call them in Cape May a "sea puss." Now everyone calls them rip currents and he said, "Here comes one!" I didn't know what he was talking about.

Anyway, he said we're going to have a rescue here. I said, "What are you talking about?" Guess what — we went out. We had rock jetties at the time in Cape May before they pumped the sand in and we went around that jetty. Was I scared? Yeah, I guess so, but my partner was so good and in fact we had a set up at that time in Cape May. We had a little stand about three foot high. We had a spool on the back of it with rope and then we had a diamond shaped can and it was attached to this spool. And we went out and we had a captain who was a fanatic that wherever you went you took that spool. In today's lifeguarding, it's entirely different, but everyone still has spools that they use in different ways, which is good because it's a lot better today.

But anyway, out we go. We exhausted the three hundred feet of line we had in there and we were in a section that if we were lucky someone would help pull us in. But no one helped. We ended going around the stone jetty. The only thing I worried about was the waves throwing us against the jetty.

Everything worked out, but that was my first rescue. We went around that jetty. We got everyone out just fine. I will give Cape May credit to this day that Cape May has never had a drowning while lifeguards were on duty. I don't know if any other town, city, or area can own up to that. I don't work for Cape May anymore — I'm retired from there.

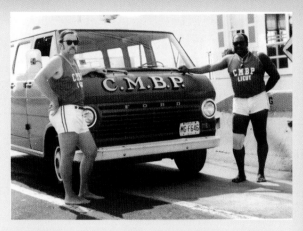

Jack Schellenger (left) is pictured outside Cape May Beach Patrol Headquarters with veteran lifeguard Ron Owens. Cape May lifeguards are always pictured with their shirts or tank tops, a requirement since the establishment of the Beach Patrol in 1911. When guards are off the stand, they must wear shirts! *Courtesy of Jack Schellenger.*

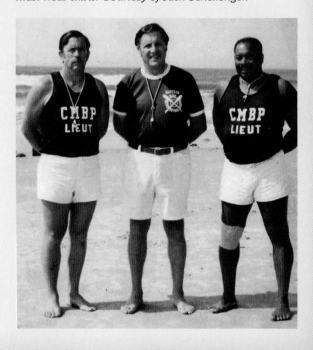

Lieutenant Jack Schellenger (left) is pictured with Cleto Cannone and Ron Owens. When this photo was taken in the 1960s the three collectively had 150 years of lifeguarding experience. *Courtesy of Jack Schellenger.*

Harry Hoehn
Interviewed March 22, 2009

Long time lifeguard legend and Allenhurst resident Harry Hoehn established his mark along the North Shore of Monmouth County. Born in 1930, his guarding roots date to his rookie year in 1947 at Eighth Avenue in Asbury Park where he worked under the tutelage of Johnny Baine. After his father "volunteered" him, Harry spent the next twenty-five summers in Allenhurst after which he moved one community north to Loch Arbor from 1970 through 1977 to take over lifeguard operations there.

Harry eventually moved into pool operations in 1978 at Ocean Township as the opening manager. Along with his long-time commitment to ocean lifeguarding, Harry also had an entrepreneurial side, owning and operating the North Channel Marina in Belmar and the Deal Lake Yacht Club restaurant in Allenhurst.

Harry has been a long time competitor in lifeguard tournaments as a rower and has participated in many competitions. He continues as a judge in many of the local tournaments and is a familiar sight at most every Monmouth County competition. Presently he is a retired college Professor of Physical Education at Queens College, part of the CUNY system in Flushing Meadows, New York.

Harry also served in the Army, joining in 1954. While stationed in Okinawa, his assignment was most appropriate — lifeguard training! In 1992, he again returned to lifeguarding in Asbury Park where he continues to this day, now as a volunteer. All in all, Harry worked thirty-six years as a paid guard during which his crews rescued thousands of people, certainly establishing his legacy in ocean guarding.

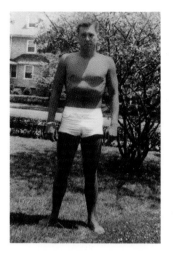

Rookie lifeguard and now lifeguard legend Harry Hoehn in 1947. The photo, taken in black and white was hand colored by his mother! *Courtesy of Harry Hoehn.*

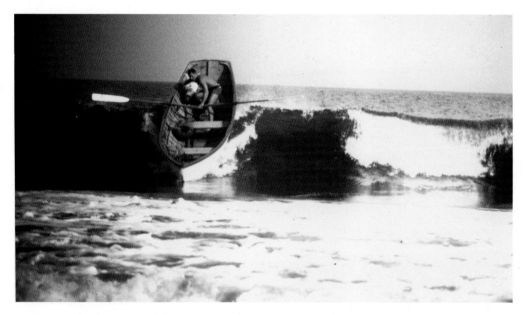

Harry Hoehn boat surfs a Hankins Skiff on an incoming wave during his early years lifeguarding. He claims he made it straight to shore after the boat leveled out! *Photo by Bob Prisco. Courtesy of Harry Hoehn.*

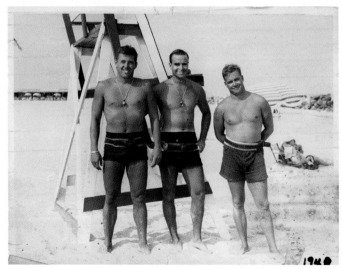

Lifeguard Harry Hoehn, left, on the beach in Asbury Park in 1948. Notice the canvas suits and canvas and leather rescue belts. *Courtesy of Harry Hoehn.*

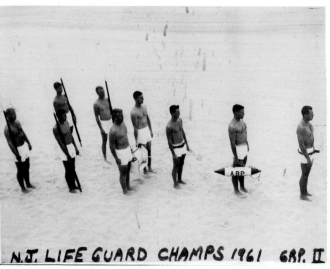

Allenhurst lifeguards were group II (smaller beach) lifeguard champs in 1961. They are pictured here marching in formation on to the beach in Asbury Park as was the tradition in the day. *Courtesy of Harry Hoehn.*

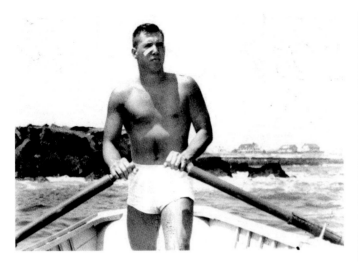

Harry Hoehn at the oars of a Hankins surfboat.
Courtesy of Harry Hoehn.

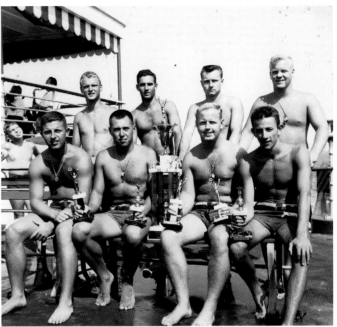

Harry Hoehn, seated, second from left and his Allenhurst beach patrol display their trophies. That summer they all donated two days wages to send one of their colleagues who couldn't afford tuition to law school. Their benevolence was covered in local newspapers. *Courtesy of Harry Hoehn.*

Rescuing 13 People at Once
Harry Hoehn, Allenhurst Beach Patrol

In 1953, a bunch of hurricanes went by. Like every week a hurricane went by because we actually canceled all the lifeguard tournaments. Every time they scheduled a tournament, we never had it because the surf was so horrendous. Every time they scheduled it, they had to cancel it. It was right at the end of the season, right after Labor Day and there were these fifteen footers. The ocean was glassy and these waves were just humungous. Everybody had gone back to school or stopped lifeguarding because they earned the maximum amount; I think it was $650 and then your father couldn't take you off his income tax anymore as a dependent. So I'm the only one left and they hired a local guy without saying anything named Frank Clifford. Nice guy, but not a very good swimmer, and not very athletic. We came down and raked the beach. We set the beach up and he said, "I forgot lunch. Can I take fifteen minutes and run home and get it?" He only lived like two blocks away. So he left right around noontime and I didn't see him again until about 3:00 in the afternoon. Fortunately I saw him at a distance because I would have killed him had I saw him close up.

Some time in the afternoon, two of my football teammates from Trenton State who worked down in Margate came up to say "hello." Kids were getting ready to go back to school and Rita Morgan had about ten girlfriends down and they all went and got in the ocean and the next thing I know I got a rip current and thirteen people were going out. I had a kid in the water who was the fastest swimmer in all of New England

prep schools named Dave Dickson — he lived right down the street in Allenhurst. He was already in the water trying to ride some of the smaller waves, so I told the two guys on the beach —and one guy was a tackle about 270 pounds — "I'm going to go out and swim past all these people and when I get out past them, I'm going to get the last couple and when I wave, pull me in." So I went past and I kept going and said, "Put your hand around the line, but don't hold on to it so I can keep going." I don't know what they did, but I just kept going. Eventually I got out and I ended up on top of this wave. I just made this wave and I'm looking back at the beach and I'm as high as the parking lot at the end of Corlies Avenue. It was a west wind and it's whipping the foam off the top of this wave and I'm saying to myself, "What the hell am I doing out here?" I kept going, and I got the last two people and I saw Davey Dickson and said, "Follow me and if anyone falls off, grab them and stick them back on the line." So I started to swim in, half dragging two girls with me and another girl is hanging on my neck and Davey's following us and finally the girl hanging on my neck let go and he grabs her, and they pulled us in. We got in just about to the pole line when this set got us. Everybody kind of washed up on the beach. The two guys from Margate waded in their clothes and pulled people up. The one girl — Davey was still coming in with her when they got caught in one of the big waves coming in and he lost her in a big wave, but he got in and the girl's rolling around out there someplace. We're looking and looking and all of a sudden about ten feet away from me I see a hand waving and we got all thirteen back on the beach. That scared the hell out of me. That was maybe the scariest rescue of my career.

The Boyd Family

The 1987 Seaside Heights annual publication lists nine Boyds, so it truly is a family affair with Hugh, Jr., Jay, John, John, Jr., Joseph, Joseph, Jr., Michael, Steven and Thomas. This story is about three veteran members of the staff but certainly the family has established a mark as super heroes of ocean rescue along the south Jersey shoreline.

By 1989, Captain John J. Boyd had been Captain of the beach patrol for sixty years! He captured the respect and admiration of his lifeguard crew. An All-American football player at Temple University where he played in the first Sugar Bowl game, he served in the Navy during WW II as captain in charge of air-sea rescues. Lifeguarding was a natural for John. During the "off" season, he was a teacher and football coach at Atlantic City High School.

Captain John Boyd's classic "Knowledge is Power" essay appeared annually in the Seaside Heights lifeguard yearbook. In that essay he espoused, "it is important that you bear in mind . . . that each rescue is a matter of life and death. You must be able to go from total relaxation to total stress instantly ... Ninety percent of our job is prevention and anticipation, backed up by experience and knowledge." The "Boyd System of Lifeguarding" invariably accounts for a perfect record — no drowning fatalities — during his tenure as captain.

As written by his wife Slim, "Lest we forget Junie 'The Man' Boyd, a giant to all who knew him and loved him for his endless efforts in projecting a family image to Seaside Heights — whether it be in education, family life, and above all, 'a Seaside Heights Lifeguard'." Hugh J. "Junie" Boyd, Jr. was a lifeguard at Seaside Heights for forty-two years, having joined the beach patrol in 1944. He followed his brothers Captain John J. Boyd and the late lieutenant Joseph J. Boyd. He was promoted to lieutenant in 1949 and assistant beach patrol captain in 1974. Junie enjoyed success within the community, becoming Superintendent of Schools in Seaside Heights where the Hugh J. Boyd, Jr. Elementary School bears his namesake.

Lifeguard Lieutenant Joseph Boyd guarded in Seaside Heights up until 1971 for a total of twenty-seven years. He died the following year at age 51 and the Joseph J. Boyd Memorial Award for Outstanding Lifeguard commemorates his legacy. His career path paralleled his brother John's, as Joe attended Temple University and served in WW II as a flight instructor. He taught in Atlantic City as well coaching football and track.

The legacy established by the Boyd's has established the Seaside Heights Beach Patrol as one of the most respected and successful beach patrols in the world. Perhaps John Boyd said it best when he wrote "A real lifeguard is a combination of brains and brawn with a great sense of personal honor."

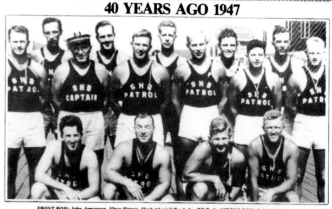

40 YEARS AGO 1947

FRONT ROW: John Armstrong, Vince Harvey, Hugh "Junie" Boyd, Jr., Bill Beale. MIDDLE ROW: Robert Young, Captain John Boyd, Joe Boyd, Whitey Paskowitz, Richard McCrea, Bob Beale. BACK ROW: Roy Borton, Chuck Kaufman, B. Casler, Unknown, Bill Arden.

Seaside Heights 1947 team photo pictures the three Boyd brothers — John and Joseph in the middle row, second and third from left, and Junie in the bottom row, second from right. *Courtesy of Steve Healey.*

Captain John J. Boyd put in sixty years lifeguarding at Seaside Heights. *Courtesy of Steve Healey.*

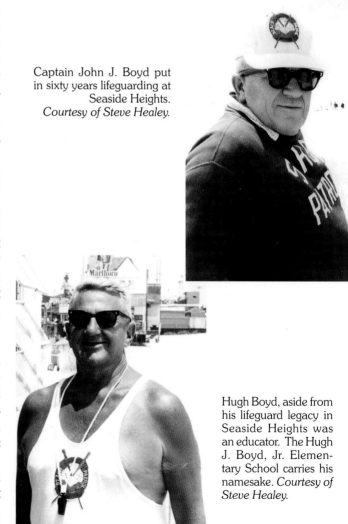

Hugh Boyd, aside from his lifeguard legacy in Seaside Heights was an educator. The Hugh J. Boyd, Jr. Elementary School carries his namesake. *Courtesy of Steve Healey.*

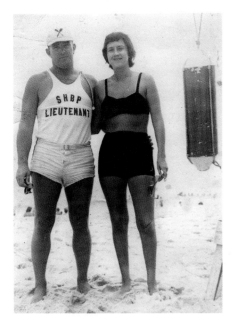

Seaside Heights Lieutenant Joseph Boyd is pictured with his wife in 1955. *Courtesy of Steve Healey.*

Rescue Beneath the Pier
Steve Healey, Seaside Heights Lifeguard

It was on a late afternoon in July 1971 that I experienced an ocean rescue crisis — the likes of which I had never experienced before or since. It all happened near the Casino Pier in Seaside Heights, New Jersey, from Sumner to Grand Avenues. As the afternoon progressed, a strong south rip current developed much more rapidly than usual resulting in large numbers of unsuspecting bathers being swept out to sea. I had witnessed and participated in many rescues in my years as a lifeguard but none that can compare to this in scope and ferocity. The rip currents became so violent from south to north that it swept nearly all the bathers under the pier. Captain John Boyd closed all the beaches as every available lifeguard in Seaside Heights became involved in this rescue. It went on for what seemed forever, lasting between one and a half to two hours involving nearly one hundred potential victims. It pitted sheer chaos and panic against the cold, calm professionalism of seasoned ocean lifesavers.

Conditions continued to deteriorate as huge waves catapulted guards and patrons alike up underneath and against the pier boardwalk and catwalks with their exposed electrical and plumbing facilities. With each receding wave brought other dangers such as being scoured against the barnacled encrusted pilings. The seasoned veterans organized and coordinated the rescues. Men such as Bob Omert made big swims and rescues aided by Erik Jersted and Ken Reed. Lt. Hugh Boyd had a girl and boy hanging on him at the same time as he clung to a pipe finally jetting each to safety on a pier catwalk with an incoming wave. I pulled numerous people to safety under the pier and on my third trip out we were told that people were in trouble at the end of the pier. We all went out time and time again until everyone was safe back on the beach.

As the sun set, we left the beach with the satisfaction of knowing that not a single life was lost and that we had added a small page to the distinguished record of the Seaside Heights Beach Patrol. That achievement was one of never losing a life while the guards were on duty — a record that stands to this day. Immediately after the beach was closed, everyone headed to "Good Time Charlie's," one of our favorite after-hours gathering spots. It was owned by Jim O'Donnell's family; O'Donnell was one of our lifeguards who had assisted in this spectacular event. Everyone earned, "A job well done!"

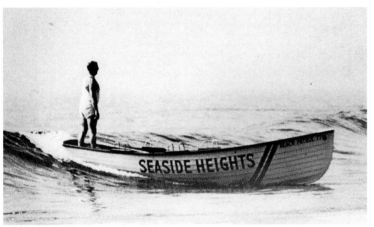

A daring Junie surfs the Van Duyne in a classic archival photo. Although this might look incredibly risky to non-lifeguards, it is relatively easy for a boatman with years of experience in the surf. *Courtesy of Steve Healey.*

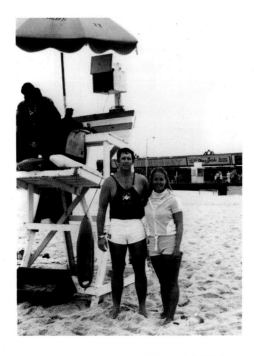

Lifeguard legend Steve Healey of Seaside Heights is pictured here with his wife Jackie in 1970. Jackie is a relative to the Boyd Brothers. *Courtesy of Steve Healey.*

Sea Girt Lifeguards Rescue 15 from the Morro Castle

Condensed from an article by Bill Dunn
of the Sea Girt Lighthouse

September 8, 1934 was the Saturday following Labor Day; the unofficial end of summer and a nor'easter was pounding the coast. People along the shore woke with foreboding to the sounds of blaring whistles and sirens as police, fire and first-aid squads responded to the first reports of a passenger ship engulfed in fire three miles off the coast of Sea Girt.

The ship was the Ward's Line T.E.L. (Turbo-Electric Liner) *Morro Castle*, a sleek, fast cruise ship on its 174th return voyage from Havana, only hours away from its scheduled docking in New York City.

Instinctively, Sea Girt's lifeguards from all over town raced to the beach at Chicago Boulevard where equipment was stored. This was the main beach by the old pavilion. In all six lifeguards arrived sometime around 7 o'clock a.m.

The nor'easter was pounding the beaches with seven to eight-foot high waves that were crashing far out in quick succession.

The Sea Girt lifeguards tried repeatedly and unsuccessfully to launch a lifeboat. But the breakers were too high, too powerful and coming too quickly for the guards to get the lifeboat past the waves.

The guards had to rely on themselves and each other in their coordinated rescues. They were encouraged and helped by many local residents who had lined the boardwalk and more that spread out along the water's edge. Head lifeguard Jack Hothusen later wrote of the "thousands of people along the shore."

Everyone was scanning the water for survivors. Ocean liners and freighters picked up the *Morro Castle's* SOS and steamed to the stricken ship and launched their own lifeboats. Coast Guard cutters were running search patterns.

Of the twelve lifeboats aboard the Morro Castle, only six made it to shore.

With fire aboard raging and making access to half the lifeboats impossible, many passengers and crew jumped overboard three miles from land. They drifted to shore carried by the currents, strong winds and large storm swells.

The first survivors, who were not picked up by fishing boats and other ships, came into sight a half-mile off Sea Girt around 9 a.m. according to news reports. They were wearing the bulky canvas lifejackets with eight cork panels. They were usually alone or in small clusters of two or three.

As a survivor was spotted, the Sea Girt lifeguards raced into the water. A guard would swim to the survivor, calm the person and get control. At that point the guard with a line attached to his leather-over-canvas lifeguard belt was pulled back to shore by the other lifeguards and volunteers who joined the effort.

Head lifeguard Jack Holthusen wrote in the 1934 issue of his national fraternity magazine, the *Circle of Zeta Psi*:

"The Coast Guards tried to launch a boat, but were swept right back in again. So our lifeguard crew waited 'till victims were just outside the line of breakers and them swam out to get them. Two of us made it.

"The first were a man and wife and a girl whom they had met in the water ... about an hour later in almost the same spot we brought in the mother of the girl. After the first job they came in singly but even at that we had very few breathing spells."

Lifeguard Tom Black told the *Asbury Park Press* on the 50th anniversary of the disaster: "We had to get to them before they were thrown with force on the beach, which would have killed them in their weakened condition. In some cases, though, we were too late."

Once on shore, the rescued were given first aid on the beach. Those needing further medical attention were taken to area hospitals. Those in good condition were taken to homes in Sea Girt and surrounding towns where they were fed, given a bed, and a telephone to call worried family and friends.

By early afternoon, when the last rescue was completed, the Sea Girt lifeguards had saved the lives of fifteen people.

In all, 137 people died as a result of the *Morro Castle* disaster, but more than four hundred survived due to the heroism of shore residents along the coast who risked their own lives to save others.

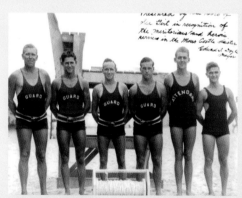

Six Sea Girt Lifeguards rescued fifteen people from the *Morro Castle,* which caught fire and came to rest off Asbury Park in September 1934. Left to right are Jack Holthusen, Tom Black, Elvin "Toots" Lake, Dick Tucker, George Braender, and Jack Little. *Courtesy of the Sea Girt Lighthouse.*

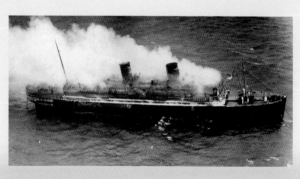

Chapter Eight

Lifeguard Tournaments

One of the most colorful and exciting pageants along the Jersey Shore are lifeguard tournaments that abound each summer. Here lifeguard crews pit their skills against other teams to demonstrate their prowess in swimming, lifesaving, rowing, running, paddling, and kayaking. It also gives them bragging rights.

These tournaments or tourneys are not new, dating back to swimming and rowing competitions against other bathhouse squads and easily date back to the nineteenth century. They are exciting to watch, especially as the surfboats blast through waves on the way out and boat surf coming back in. Great skill is necessary to manage the three hundred-pound boats through the surf. They also demonstrate the skill necessary to become a lifeguard. The oldest continuously run tournament in New Jersey is held each summer in Ocean Grove.

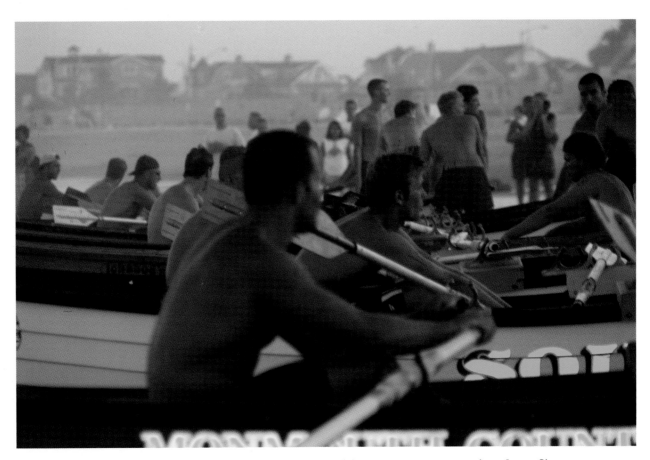

Lifeguard rowing teams await the drop of the starter's flag in one of the exciting tournaments along Jersey Shore. *Courtesy of Nancy Kegelman.*

The perceptions held by some lifeguard crews and among the laity often mirror the erroneous notion that the winners of competitions offer the public the best protection. While not diminishing the necessity of athletic prowess, competition focuses on the many skills that ensure the public's safety. This does not necessarily mean they are more conscientious lifeguards.

Some competitors specialize in events and train for many seasons to master the skills necessary to compete in their event. Some rowing crews train all winter to prep for the busy summer competitive season.

Periodically the National Lifeguard tournaments sponsored by the United States Lifesaving Association come to New Jersey and are held at Cape May. The Monmouth County team has never scored lower than third place in this event and won the national competition in 1983. At the nationals, hundreds of guards from throughout the United States compete with the "winningest" team from Los Angeles County.

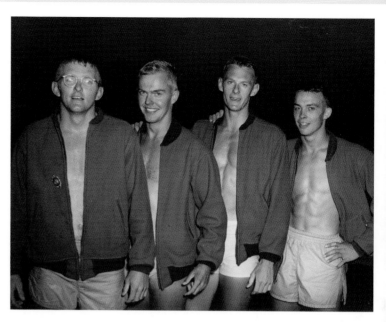

The winners of the first annual Surf Dash Event in South Jersey (left to right) Morgan H. Lear, Jr., Bob Ditmars, Dick Mendenhall, and David (last name unknown) were from Stone Harbor Beach Patrol. It was held in Sea Isle City in 1949. Today, their sixty-person beach patrol guards Stone Harbor's 2.3 miles of beach. *Courtesy of Captain Sandy Bosacco.*

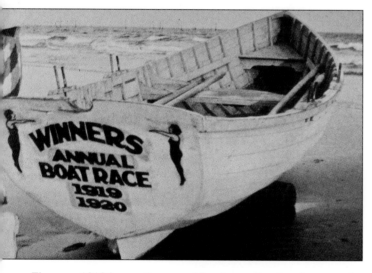

The year 1919 began the annual boating and swimming races for the championship of the Atlantic City Beach Patrol. The swimming champions were Fred Estergren and Owan Kertland.

Lifeguard tournaments date back to rivalries between hotel crews. Lavallette did win their 1939 tournament, publicized by this poster. *Courtesy of Gordon Hesse.*

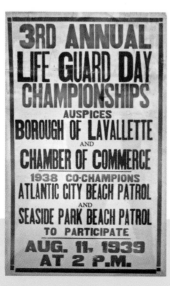

3RD ANNUAL LIFE GUARD DAY CHAMPIONSHIPS
AUSPICES
BOROUGH OF LAVALLETTE
AND
CHAMBER OF COMMERCE
1938 CO-CHAMPIONS
ATLANTIC CITY BEACH PATROL
AND
SEASIDE PARK BEACH PATROL
TO PARTICIPATE
AUG. 11, 1939 AT 2 P.M.

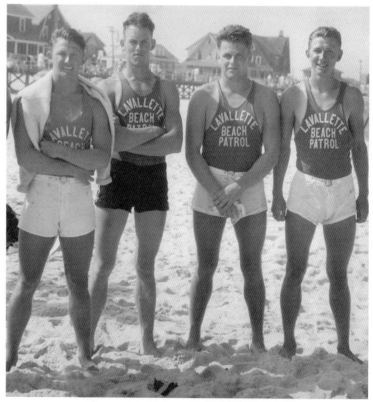

The 1939 Lavallette Beach Patrol was titled "Atlantic Coast Lifeguard Champions" following the tournament. They competed against various East Coast lifeguards from New York City to Miami. Left to right are Rudy Krone, Harry Bloom, Elmer Brackman, and Al Krone. *Courtesy of Gordon Hesse.*

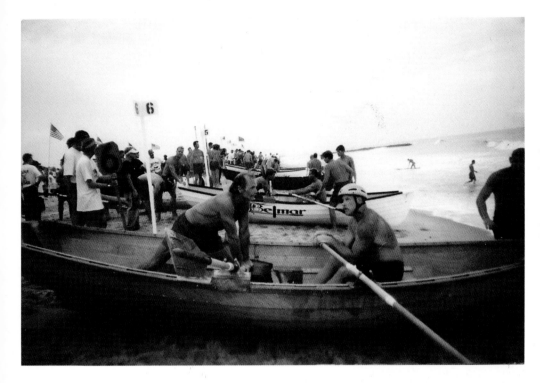

Tournaments are filled with anticipation of the event as well as the aura and pageantry of the entire competition scene. Here rowers await the starter's signal. The stand-up/sit-down configuration gives great control to the rowers. *Courtesy of John McCahill.*

United States Lifesaving Association 2008 national rowing champion Bill George (obscured by water in the bow seat) from Monmouth Beach breaks through a wave in an Asay constructed self-bailing surfboat. His rowing partner is Chris Hock from Fort Lauderdale. The team scored in first place. All water taken aboard quickly drains through holes which sit just above the waterline. *Courtesy of Bill George.*

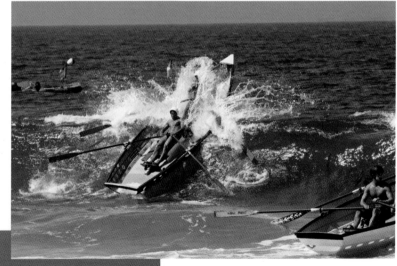

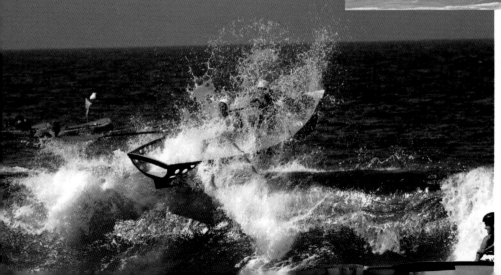

As their boat tops the wave, it is almost completely airborne highlighting both the force of the wave and the power of the rowers. *Courtesy of Bill George.*

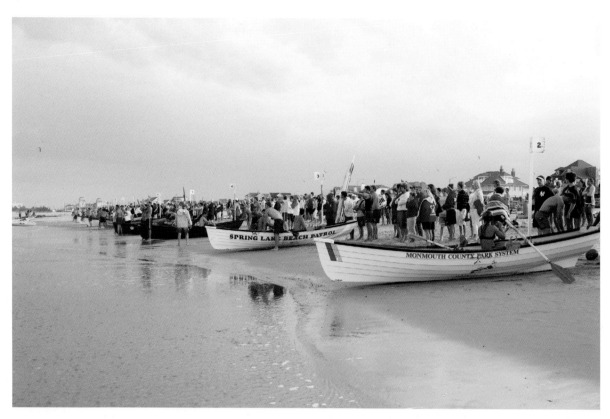

The events are festive, colorful, and draw large crowds. Most crews sponsor "after parties" to celebrate the event, with all teams invited. This is the 2009 Jersey Shore Lifeguard Relays, first run in 1975. At that time, it was the largest tournament in New Jersey with fifteen teams participating. It has since been scaled back.

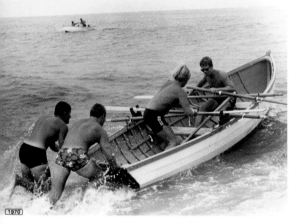

This 1970s photo shows a Hankin's skiff launched during a tournament in Avon-by-the-Sea. Rowers are Spike Fowler in the bow, Bill Lynch in the stern, and launchers John Sosdian and George Herbert.

Boating collisions in heavy surf are inevitable as an intense moment unfolds during a south Jersey competition in 1985. The surfboats are Van Duyne skiffs. *Courtesy of Buzz Mogck.*

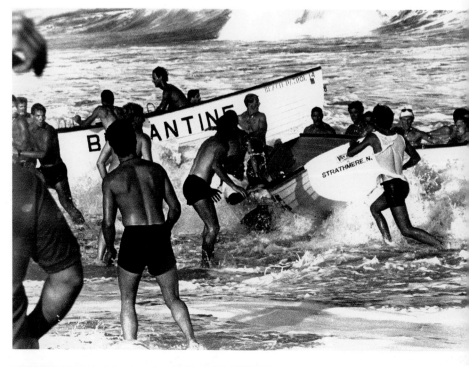

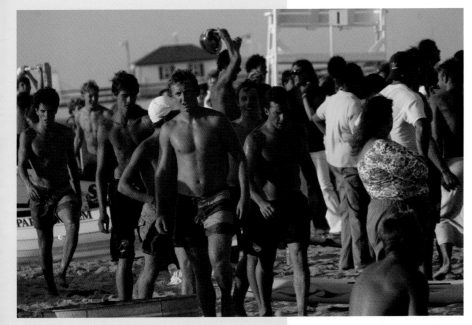

Events draw large crowds of lifeguard competitors as well as spectators. *Courtesy of Nancy Kegelman*

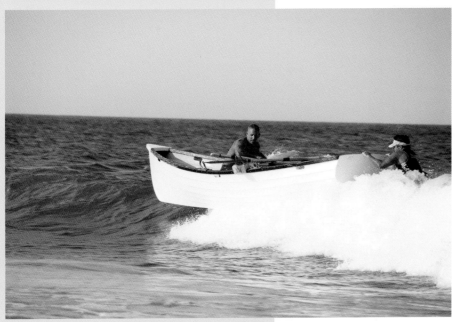

A boat crew hangs on a wave during the 2009 Jersey Shore Lifeguard Relays, held in Avon-by-the-Sea.

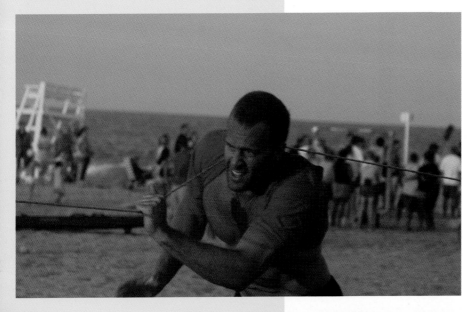

Grit and determination are necessary ingredients to win in the line rescue event. Offshore is a competitor "victim" who has been rescued by a lifeguard attached to the line. Both will be pulled in. *Courtesy of Nancy Kegelman.*

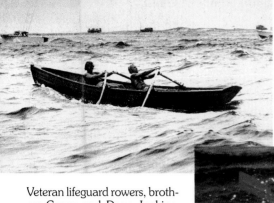

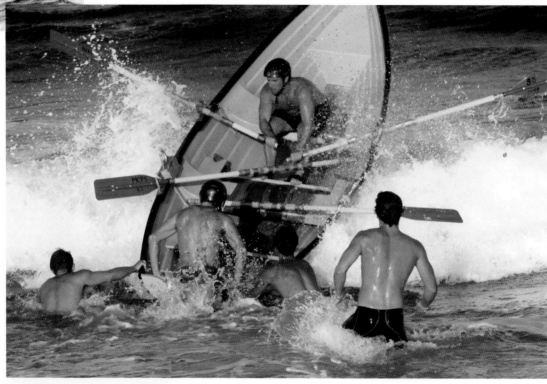

Veteran lifeguard rowers, brothers Comp and Dave Jenkins, won this 1978 championship ten-mile row in Long Beach Island, beating their nearest rivals by half a mile. The two dominated rowing events for years. The bend in the oars shows the power of their rowing stroke. *Courtesy of Harry Dowian, Asbury Park Press.*

Surfboat challenges take spirit and skill to steer the three hundred-pound boats through the waves. *Courtesy of Nancy Kegelman.*

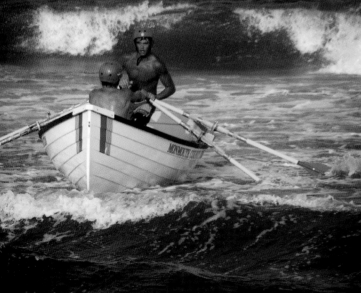

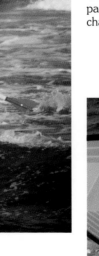

Generally speaking, going out is the easy part. Landing the surfboat safely is a real challenge. *Courtesy of Nancy Kegelman.*

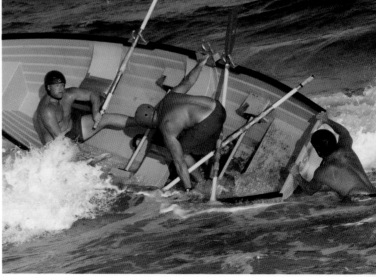

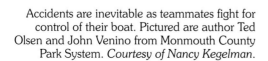

Accidents are inevitable as teammates fight for control of their boat. Pictured are author Ted Olsen and John Venino from Monmouth County Park System. *Courtesy of Nancy Kegelman.*

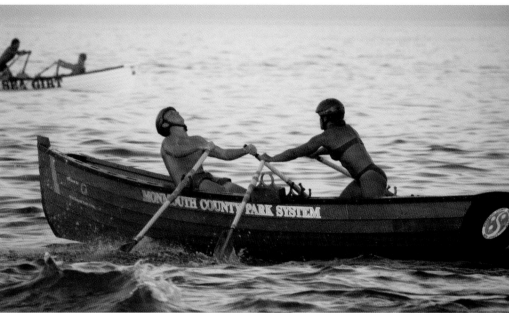

Lifeguards in Monmouth County New Jersey are the only crews left in the United States to still use the standup "boating" style of rowing. This method gives superior control and steering of the boat, and certainly takes lots to training to master this unique skill. *Courtesy of Nancy Kegelman.*

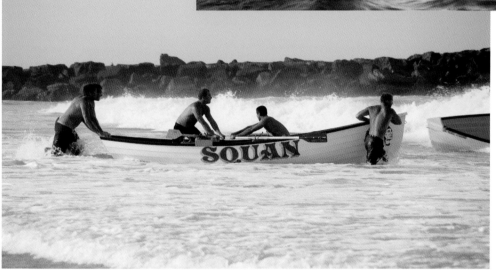

Rowing an Asay fiberglass surfboat, the crew from Manasquan battles the surf during the Jersey Shore Lifeguard Relays.

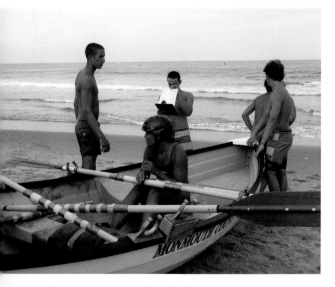

Female competitor Michelle Tomaino, a national rowing champion awaits the start of her event while the tournament captain checks the rules. *Courtesy of Nancy Kegelman.*

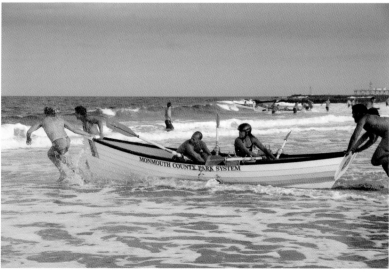

A very rare husband and wife boat crew, B. Michael and Michelle Tomaino, are launched into the surf during the 2009 Jersey Shore Lifeguard Relays. Both are USLA national champions.

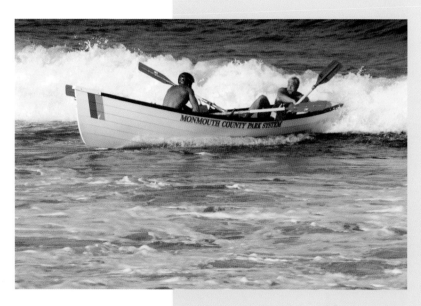

Incoming boats on waves are difficult to keep from sheering and broaching. A skilled crew however can surf the boat straight to shore. Author Ted Olsen is in the stern. *Courtesy of Nancy Kegelman.*

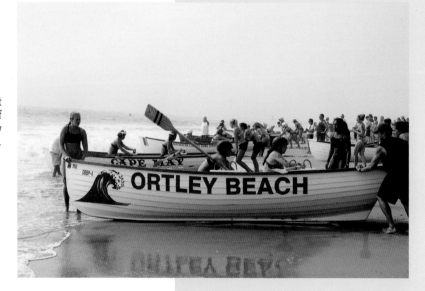

Rowers in the All Women Tournament prepare for a launch through the surf at the 2009 event hosted by Gateway National Recreation at Sandy Hook.

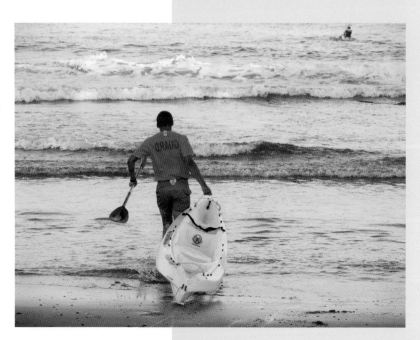

Rescue kayaks, lightweight and fast are relatively new competitive watercraft. They have been used along the Jersey Shore since the 1980s. *Courtesy of Nancy Kegelman.*

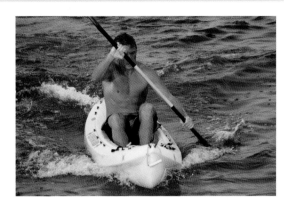
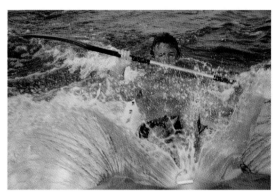

Kayaks are far easier to control and maneuver than surfboats and, in many places, have almost replaced boats as the rescue craft of choice. Despite their lack of heritage and tradition, they are faster, less expensive, and easier to maintain. *Courtesy of Nancy Kegelman.*

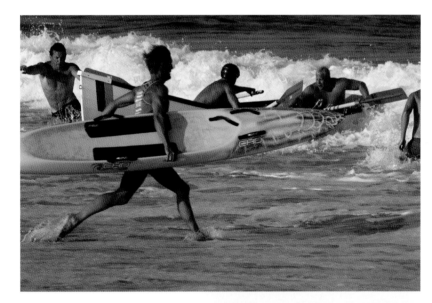

There is never a lack of action in lifeguard tournaments. Pictured is author Ted Olsen in the stern. *Courtesy of Nancy Kegelman.*

Team paddleboard events are exciting, especially in heavy surf conditions. *Courtesy of Nancy Kegelman.*

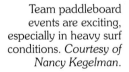
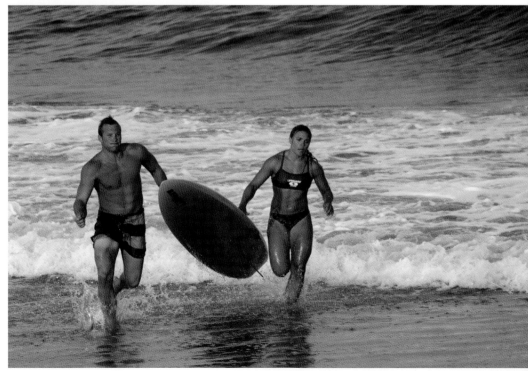

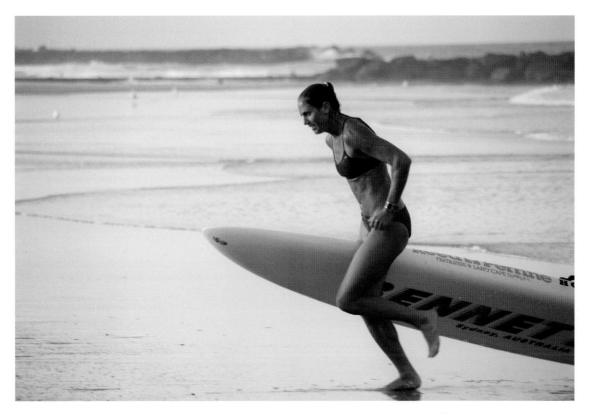

Most lifeguard events now require female participation. This was unheard of in the male dominated sport up until the 1990s. Competitive females easily keep up with and often defeat their male counterparts in swimming and paddling events.

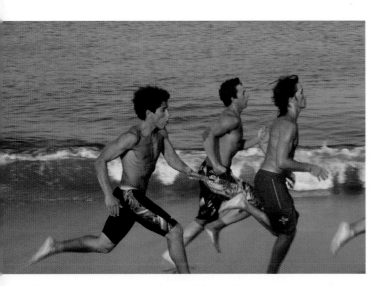

Running is a major part of ocean lifeguarding as guards may have to race to a distant location to reach their victims. Pictured are guards sprinting in the hard sand near the water's edge. *Courtesy of Nancy Kegelman.*

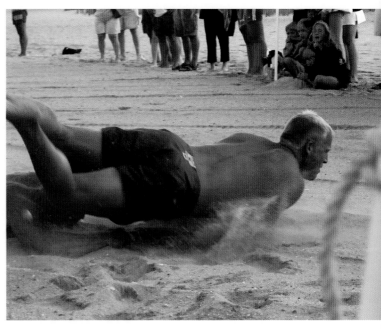

One running event is "beach flags." Very much like musical chairs, there is one less flag than the number of competitors with one lifeguard eliminated each round. It is a rough and tumble event and brings out the stamina and heart in competitors. Pictured: author Ted Olsen dives for a flag. *Courtesy of Nancy Kegelman.*

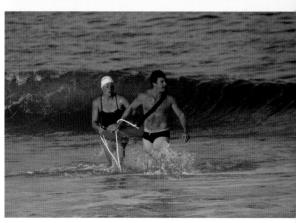

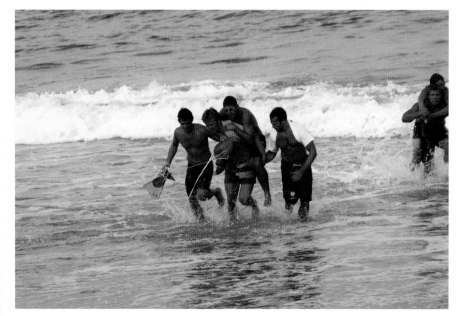

Events consisting of practice rescues are excellent demonstrations to the public on how quickly lifeguards must react. *Courtesy of Nancy Kegelman.*

In some rescue events, the competitor rescuers must carry the competitor "victim" from the water to the finish line. *Courtesy of Nancy Kegelman.*

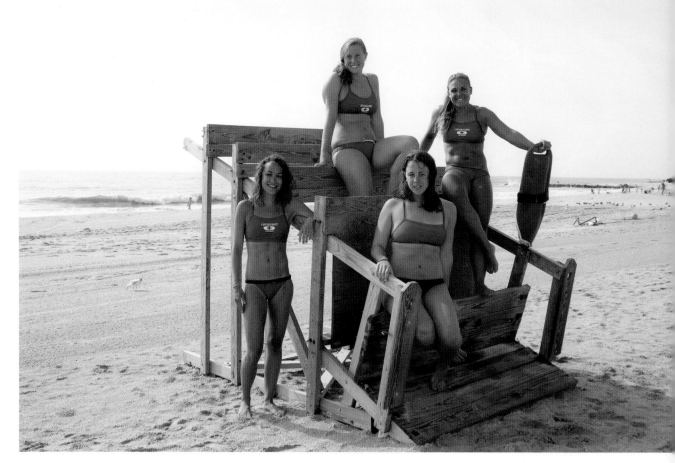

2009 Winners of the Division 1 All Women's Lifeguard Tournament held at Gateway National Recreation Area at Sandy Hook. The females from Monmouth County Park System have won this championship for the past ten years in a row. Pictured, left to right, are: Elizabeth Luick, Jordan Crosby, Taylor Crosby, and Michelle Tomaino.

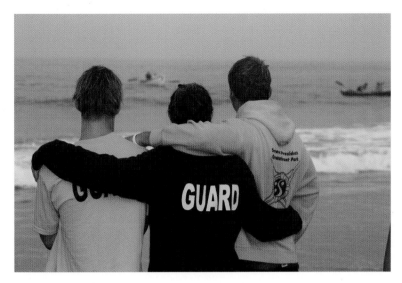

Lifeguarding becomes a way of life that establishes lifetime fellowships. *Courtesy of Nancy Kegelman.*

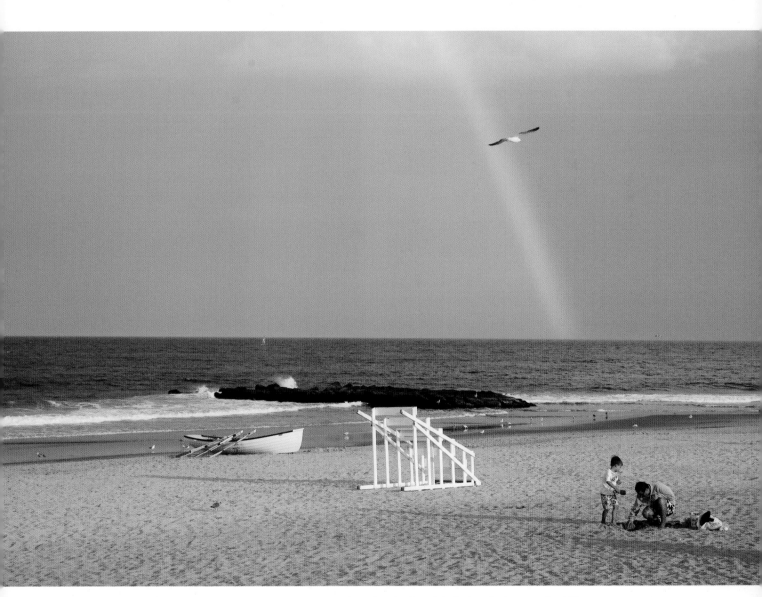

This could be the lucky end of the day for these beachgoers in Avon-by-the-Sea. Might they find a pot of gold?

Bibliography

Applegate, Lloyd R. *Life of Service: William Augustus Newell*. Ocean County, New Jersey: Ocean County Historical Society, 1994.

Atlantic City Beach Patrol Benevolent Organization. *A Brief Sketch of the Atlantic City Beach Patrol*. Atlantic City, New Jersey: Atlantic City Beach Patrol Benevolent Organization, 1956.

Atlantic City Life Guards Beneficial Association. *Souvenir Book*. Atlantic City, New Jersey: Atlantic City Life Guards Beneficial Association, 1918.

Barnett, J.P. *The Lifesaving Guns of David Lyle*. South Bend, Indiana: South Bend Replicas, Inc., 1974.

Brewster, B. Chris (editor). *Open Water Lifesaving: The United States Lifesaving Association Manual*. Upper Saddle River, New Jersey: Brady/Prentice-Hall, Inc., 2003.

Butler, Frank. *Book of the Boardwalk*. Atlantic City, New Jersey: Haines and Company, 1952.

Cunningham, John T. and Kenneth D. Cole. *Atlantic City: Images of America*. Charleston, South Carolina: Arcadia Publishing, 2000.

English, A.L. *History of Atlantic City*. Philadelphia, Pennsylvania: Dickson and Gilling Publishers, 1884.

"Entertaining a Nation: The Career of Long Branch." *Schenck's Guide*. Bayonne, New Jersey: Jersey Printing Company, 1940.

Fernicola, Dr. Richard G. *Twelve Days of Terror*. Guilford, Connecticut: The Lyons Press, 2001.

Funnell, Charles E. *By the Beautiful Sea: The Rise and High Times of the Great American Resort, Atlantic City*. New Brunswick, New Jersey: Rutgers University Press, 1983.

Gensch, Delores M. *Avon-by-the-Sea: Images of America*. Charleston, South Carolina: Arcadia Publishing, 2000.

Gibbons, Richard F. and Florence. *Lifesaving Stories: Written and Oral History*. Flyer, no date.

Guthorn, Dr. Peter J. *Sea Bright Skiff and Other Jersey Shore Boats*. New Brunswick, New Jersey: Rutgers University Press, 1971.

Hesse, Gordon. *All Summer Long: Tales and Lore of Lifeguarding on the Atlantic*. Bay Head, New Jersey: Jersey Shore Publications, 2005.

Judge, M.D., Walter F. *The Spring Lake Lifeguard Spanning 100 Years, 1906 – 2006: A Pictorial Compendium*. Spring Lake, New Jersey: Carl Steets Publisher, 2006.

Kobbe, Gustave. *Jersey Coast and Pines*. Short Hills, New Jersey: self-published, 1889.

Long Beach Township Beach Patrol. *Long Beach Township Beach Patrol Lifeguard Yearbook*. Long Beach, New Jersey: Long Beach Township Beach Patrol, various dates.

McMahon, William. *So Young … So Gay! Story of the Boardwalk 1870 – 1970*. Atlantic City, New Jersey: Atlantic City Press Publication, 1970.

Merryman, J. H. *The United States Life-Saving Service – 1880*. Golden, Colorado: Outbooks, 1981.

Miller, Fred. *Ocean City Beach Patrol: Images of America*. Charleston, South Carolina: Arcadia Publishing, 2004.

Moss, George Jr. and Karen L. Schnitzspahn. *Victorian Summers at the Grand Hotels of Long Branch, New Jersey*. Sea Bright, New Jersey: Ploughshare Press, 2000.

Scott, Arthur E. "Longtime Lifeguard Kept Shore Safe for Half Century." *Asbury Park Press*, August 29, 2005.

Seaside Heights Lifeguard Association Annual Publications, 1982-1987

Shanks, Ralph, Wick York, and Lisa Woo Shanks. *U.S. Life-Saving Service, Rescues and Architecture of the Early Coast Guard*. Petaluma, California: Costaño Books, 1996.

Wilson, Harold F. *The Jersey Shore: A Social and Economic History of the Counties of Atlantic, Cape May, Monmouth, and Ocean*. New York, New York: Lewis Historical Publishing Company, Inc., 1953.

The Story of the Jersey Shore: New Jersey Historical Series, Vol. 4. Princeton, New Jersey: D. Van Nostrand Company, 1964.

Online Resources

~ Avalon's Past: avalonspast.com
~ Long Beach Township Lifeguards: lbtbp.com
~ North Wildwood Beach Patrol: wildwood-by-the-sea.com
~ Sea Girt Beach Patrol: seagirtbeachpatrol.org
~ Stone Harbor Beach Patrol: stone-harbor.nj.us
~ USLA.org

Index

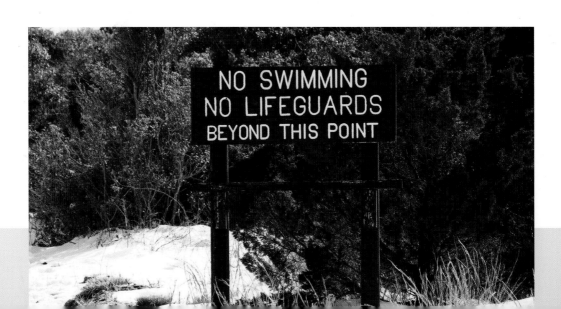